GLUCAGON
IN GASTROENTEROLOGY
AND HEPATOLOGY

Pharmacological, Clinical
and Therapeutic Implications

GLUCAGON
IN
GASTROENTEROLOGY
AND
HEPATOLOGY

PHARMACOLOGICAL, CLINICAL, AND THERAPEUTIC IMPLICATIONS

Edited by J.Picazo,M.D.

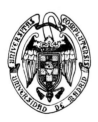

The Proceedings of an International Workshop held in Madrid on 23 October, 1981, under the auspices of the Medical School of the Universidad Complutense, Madrid.

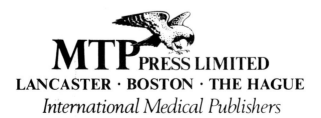

MTP PRESS LIMITED
LANCASTER · BOSTON · THE HAGUE
International Medical Publishers

Published in the UK and Europe by
MTP Press Limited
Falcon House
Lancaster, England

British Library Cataloguing in Publication Data

Glucagon in gastroenterology and hepatology.
  1. Gastroenterology—Congresses 2. Glucagon—Congresses
I. Picazo, J.
  616.3 RC817
   ISBN 0-85200-447-8

Published in the USA by
MTP Press
A division of Kluwer Boston Inc
190 Old Derby Street
Hingham, MA 02043, USA

Filmset by Speedlith Photo Litho Ltd, Manchester and printed by UPS (Blackburn) Ltd.

Contents

Glucagon in Gastroenterology and Hepatology

ERRATA: p. 22, 3rd paragraph: The question by *Diamant* should read: 'Do I understand you correctly? Is B proglucagon?'

p. 106: The sub-heading '(c) Post-sphincterotomy' should read: '(c) Post-endoscopic sphincterotomy'.

Preface

It was indeed a great pleasure for me to chair this workshop on Glucagon in Gastroenterology and Hepatology. In a way this meeting was a follow-up to one held in 1978. On that occasion the workshop participants defined the physiological role of glucagon, and discussed its uses in clinical gastroenterology, particularly as an aid to diagnosis in the areas of endoscopy and radiology. They discussed the spasmolytic effects of glucagon and its value in the treatment of biliary colic. They considered its possible hepatotrophic effect and pondered on the beneficial effect which its use might have in liver diseases.

In the years since that first meeting several issues have been clarified. The usefulness of glucagon as an aid to gastro-duodenoscopy and ERCP now seems well-established. Some exciting new developments have occurred, one of which is an assessment of the inhibitory effects of glucagon on gastric acid secretion. Some impressive work has also been done on glucagon analogues and fragments. Improved techniques in the field of endoscopy have provided an accurate means of assessing the action of glucagon on the sphincter of Oddi, and thoughts are beginning to turn to the therapeutic role which glucagon might play in sphincter of Oddi disorders. Work has also progressed on the study of liver regeneration, and results are beginning to emerge from clinical studies of the use of glucagon in certain liver diseases. Taking all these points into account, it did indeed seem time to repeat the 1978 exercise, and to hold another workshop in order to discuss some of them.

The format chosen for the meeting was the same as that of the first workshop. It was a small meeting attended only by specially invited participants, people who really had something important to say. As Professor Oriol Bosch so rightly pointed out in the preface of the proceedings of the

vii

earlier workshop (*Glucagon in Gastroenterology*, 1979, MTP Press), one of the main attractions of this type of meeting is its multi-disciplinary character. Our knowledge of medical science is such, and is growing at such a pace, that it is increasingly necessary to specialize. It is equally evident that the more we specialize, the more important it becomes for us periodically to get out of our precise, but sometimes narrow, furrows in order to take a look at our work from other angles. The value of the exchanges which take place at meetings such as this is immeasurable. It often comes, not only during the official workshop sessions, but also through the contacts made informally. It is an aspect which is reflected in a comment made at the end of one of the coffee-breaks: 'Isn't it great,' said an excited participant, 'do you know, it must be twenty years since I last had a conversation like this with a clinician'.

At the end of the workshop I expressed my thanks, as chairman, to all those who had come to Madrid, many from far distant countries, to present their views and to report their findings. With the publication of this book I should like to repeat my thanks to these people, for it is they and their contributions which made the workshop what it was. Coupled with this I must thank Dr José Picazo who organized the event, and made it possible for us all to meet. In this he was most ably assisted by Mari Carmen Hernández, and by Mariann Strid Christensen. I congratulate Dr Picazo and Pamela Freebody on the publication of this book. It was they who had to gather the manuscripts together and pull our far-ranging discussions into shape. Finally, I should like to thank our publishers for working so co-operatively to produce this book. To everyone involved, I extend my thanks for your contributions to what I feel to be a most interesting and worthwhile project.

FRANCISCO VILARDELL
Workshop Chairman

Director
Escuela de Patología Digestiva
Barcelona, April 1982   *Universidad Autónoma*

Participants

A. L. Baker
Liver Study Unit
University of Chicago
Chicago, IL 60637
USA

N. L. R. Bucher
Harvard Medical School
Massachusetts General Hospital
Shriners Burns Institute
Boston, MA 02114 USA

J. Christiansen
Kirurgisk Afdeling D Køvenhavns Amts
Sygehus 2600 Glostrup Denmark

O. Daniel
Ysbyty Glan Clwyd Rhyl, Clwyd
LL18 5UJ UK

B. Diamant
Novo Research Institute DK-2880
Bagsværd Denmark

J. D. Hardcastle
Department of Surgery University
Hospital Queen's Medical Centre
Nottingham, Notts. NG7 2UH UK

J. B. Jaspan
Department of Medicine University of
Chicago Chicago, IL 60637 USA

R. E. Miller
Department of Radiology Indiana
University Medical Center Indianapolis,
IN 46223 USA

H. Oka
First Department of Internal
 Medicine
University of Tokyo Tokyo 113 Japan

K. Okuda
First Department of Medicine Chiba
University Medical School Chiba City
280 Japan

A. Oriol-Bosch
Facultad de Medicina Universidad
Complutense Madrid 3 Spain

J.-F. Rey
Département d'Hépatologie et
 de Gastro-entérologie
Institut Arnault Tzanck 06700 Saint
Laurent du Var France

J. Skucas
Department of Radiology Rochester
University Medical Center Rochester,
NY 14642 USA

F. Vilardell
Escuela de Patología Digestiva
Universidad Autónoma Barcelona 25
Spain

ix

1

Glucagon: basic pathophysiological considerations

J. B. JASPAN

INTRODUCTION

Although at the time not clearly recognized, Banting and Best[1] were the first to describe the biological activity of glucagon. In their now famous experiments of 1921, they noted a small, transient rise in blood glucose after injection of pancreatic extract into depancreatized dogs. Soon thereafter, Kimball and Murlin[2] focused on this finding, attributing it to a hormone which they named glucagon which they proposed functioned to increase plasma glucose. Now, over 50 years later, this role has been more completely defined, with numerous recent studies essentially reinforcing this earlier observation. In addition a number of other functions and actions have been recognized.

STRUCTURE/BIOSYNTHESIS

Glucagon was subsequently isolated and found to comprise a 29 amino acid peptide of molecular weight 3485. The sequence in virtually all mammals studied is identical, although glucagons from a few aquatic species, including shark and anglerfish, exhibit slight differences in amino acid content and sequence[3]. In contrast to insulin, glucagon possesses no cysteine residues or disulphide bonds, and a specific tertiary structure has not been elucidated. The

1

structure of glucagon has been confirmed by synthesis in a number of laboratories[4]. The primary sequence is shown in Figure 1, Chapter 2, of this book.

Following the discovery of proinsulin[5], the biosynthetic precursor of insulin, biosynthetic studies on a variety of peptide hormones have indicated that the primary gene products differ substantially from the putative hormonal structure. Evidence has accumulated to suggest that a variety of larger intermediate forms of many hormones may exist, which are progressively cleaved to the final hormonal product by virtue of spontaneous or enzyme induced post-translational modifications in the cell of origin or in the plasma. Thus it has been shown that glucagon is synthesized as a larger precursor molecule which has a molecular size three to five times larger than glucagon[6]. To summarize this work, it appears that the gene product of the glucagon precursor synthesized in pancreas and gut is identical. Differences in post-translational modifications in these tissues result in a family of peptides characteristically found in each tissue. This is illustrated schematically in Figure 1. Peptide 5 is glucagon. Both tissues contain the same higher

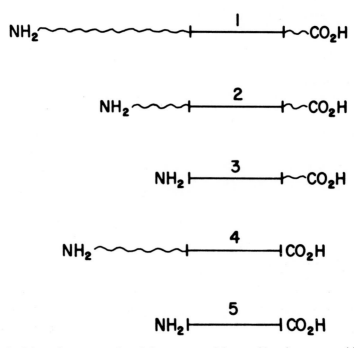

Figure 1 Schematic representation of glucagon-containing peptides of pancreas and intestine. The structure of glucagon is depicted by the straight lines and extensions on that sequence by wavy lines (Tager, H. S. and Markese, J., 1979. Reprinted, with permission, from *J. Biol. Chem.*, **254**, 2229

molecular weight peptide (peptide 1) of 12 000 mol. wt. which is thought to be the peptide known as glicentin. A 8000 mol. wt. form (peptide 2), progressively cleaved at both amino and carboxyl termini, is also present in both tissues. Peptide 3 (4500 mol. wt.) consists of glucagon with an 8 amino acid extension at the carboxyl terminus, isolated from commercially available crystalline glucagon, which is thought to be a fragment of the 9000 mol. wt. larger precursor form (peptide 4), detectable in pancreas and, in certain circumstances, in plasma. For a more detailed review the reader is referred to reference 6.

It has been suggested that the amino terminus extension sequence of proglucagon contains biologically active sequences, as has been shown for the precursor forms of ACTH, lipotropin, MSH and enkephalin. It is, however, also possible that the additional sequence represents an inactive peptide as is the C-peptide extension of insulin.

A recent study has provided evidence of transformation of glucagon-like immunoreactivity (GLI) of gut into glucagon extracellularly after injection into plasma[7]. Although of great interest and potential importance, this finding must await further confirmation.

In summary, current evidence suggests that glucagon is synthesized as a 18 000 mol. wt. precursor molecule which is progressively cleaved. predominantly intracellularly, by way of a number of intermediates, into the 3500 mol. wt. biologically active hormone. Closely related glucagon forms are detectable in gut of all species derived from the same gene but differing from precursor and intermediate forms of glucagon in pancreas by virtue of different post-synthetic modifications. A-cells in stomach and upper small bowel of dogs and other animals, identical to pancreatic A-cells, contain identical precursor and product forms of glucagon. The presence of such cells in the gut of man has not been conclusively demonstrated, nor completely excluded.

ORIGIN

Glucagon is secreted by the A (α) cells of the pancreatic islets. Careful immunohistochemical analysis by Orci and Perrelet[8] has revealed that the distribution of glucagon in islet is not uniform throughout the pancreas. Thus, islets from the dorsal aspect of the pancreas (head, body and tail) are rich in glucagon, while those in the ventral pancreas are glucagon-poor. Reciprocal localization of pancreatic polypeptide exists, while insulin and somatostatin are equally distributed in both segments. The physiological explanation of these findings is not known.

As noted above, the upper small bowel in animals in addition to GLI contains glucagon in cells indistinguishable from pancreatic A-cells[9]. Whether this is true in man is not certain[10].

Within every pancreatic islet, rather than random cell distribution, there is a distinctive anatomical arrangement of glucagon, insulin and somatostatin secreting cells (A, B and D cells). This is shown in Figure 2. B-cells are distributed in the central portion of the islet with A-cells at the periphery and D-cells at the interface. Although the explanation of this relationship has not been fully elucidated, these cells almost certainly function co-operatively, by means of intercellular connections, in determining the minute to minute fine regulation of islet secretion, as discussed below.

SECRETION

Glucagon secretion is regulated under the control of circulating, local and neurogenic factors, as summarized in Table 1. Although many factors appear to influence glucagon secretion, it is likely that under both ambient conditions

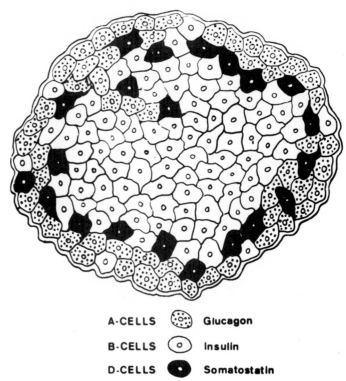

A-CELLS   Glucagon

B-CELLS   Insulin

D-CELLS   Somatostatin

Figure 2   Anatomical relationship of A, B and D cells within islets of Langerhans. (Unger, R. H. and Orci, L. 1977. Reprinted, with permission, from *Arch. Intern. Med.*, **137**, 482)

Table 1   Physiological influences in the control of glucagon secretion. Major factors are underlined

Factor	Effect on glucagon secretion
Circulating factors	
Nutrients and metabolites:	
Protein	Stimulates
–Hyperglycaemia	Suppresses
Glucose	
–Hypoglycaemia	Stimulates
Free fatty acids	Suppress*
Ketones	Suppress
Hormones:	
Insulin	Suppresses hypersecretion in diabetes
Secretin	Stimulates (pharmacologic doses)
Somatostatin	Suppresses
Cholecystokinin–Pancreozymin	Stimulates ⌉ particularly in
GIP	Stimulates ⌋ face of hypoglucaemia
[Secondary effects of these are related to blood glucose levels, e.g., insulin induced hypoglycaemia stimulates glucagon secretion, etc.]	
Local factors	
Local somatostatin and insulin	Minute-to-minute fine regulation of output A, B, D cell inter-relationship
Prostaglandin E	Stimulates
Calcium	Permissive to glucagon secretory or suppressive factors
Neurogenic factors	
Sympathetic:	
Splanchnic nerve stimulation	Stimulate
Epinephrine	
Parasympathetic:	
Nerve stimulation	??
Acetylcholine	Stimulate
Local peptidergic nerves:	
VIP	Stimulate
Tetragastrin	
Neurotensin	Stimulate; blocked by
Substance P	H$_2$ receptor antagonist

*Fat ingestion stimulates glucagon probably via release of cholecystokinin–pancreozymin

and physiological stress it is predominantly regulated by a few primary influences. These include protein (stimulatory) and glucose (suppressive). Hypoglycaemia is a powerful stimulus to glucagon secretion. Although under varying circumstances a variety of hormones can be shown to effect glucagon secretion, the most important are insulin and somatostatin (hormonal status yet to be established). However, the effects of insulin and somatostatin are primarily local or paracrine, operating within the islets by virtue of intercellular junctions. Thus, glucagon stimulates both insulin and somatostatin, somatostatin inhibits both insulin and glucagon, and insulin inhibits both somatostatin and glucagon. It is believed that hidden within this rather complex intra-islet communication system, lies the explanation of the local fine regulation of islet secretion. Disturbances in this system have been

5

suggested to underlie the abnormalities in islet secretion seen in conditions such as diabetes[11]. Extracellular calcium and intracellular calcium transport are important in regulating A-cell secretion. Calcium appears to be necessary as a permissive factor to facilitate secretory or suppressive influences, and in the absence of extracellular calcium, for example, hyperglycaemia has been shown to induce glucagon release rather than inhibition[12] in a manner reminiscent of the paradoxical glucagon response to glucose in diabetes. Of the neurogenic controls, sympathetic nervous system stimulation of glucagon secretion is the most important, in large measure accounting for the hyperglucagonaemia of stress. In the physiological response to stress, therefore, the sympathetic nervous system (and epinephrine) is pivotal and the important glucagon mediated effects are absent without epinephrine mediated glucagon release. This is seen, for example, in the autonomic neuropathy of diabetes, which may result in severe, unresponsive hypoglycaemic episodes. A number of other factors, such as prostaglandins and neurogenic peptides, have been shown to effect glucagon secretion but their roles in the overall control of glucagon secretion remain to be established.

CIRCULATING LEVELS AND PHYSIOLOGICAL RESPONSES

Normal fasting glucagon levels range from 30 to 150 pg/ml, depending on the particular antiserum used in the immunoassay. However, glucagon in normal plasma is heterogeneous, comprising a number of molecular forms of immunoreactive glucagon (IRG). These consist of a large molecular weight form, eluting in the void volume of a chromatographic column (A-peak), a 9000 mol. wt. form which is an intermediate glucagon form, as discussed above, designated peptide 4 in Figure 1 [(B-peak), barely detectable in normal plasma], the putative 3500 mol. wt. 'true' glucagon (C-peak) and a smaller than 2000 mol. wt. (D-peak) fraction, thought to be a degradative fragment[13,14]. The A and C peak components, present in variable proportions in normal plasma, comprise $>90\%$ of plasma IRG levels in plasma of healthy subjects. Elevation of the B-peak components is a hallmark of certain diseases as discussed below. Of these, only the 3500 mol. wt. fraction is biologically active or biologically responsive to stimulatory and suppressive factors, to any significant degree. Thus, in terms of biologic activity or responses, IRG components other than the C-peak component represent contamination since they are measured as part of whole plasma IRG levels but do not contribute to the physiology of the hormone. The degree to which these other components are present will compromise accurate measurement of plasma glucagon under any particular set of circumstances. Normal patterns and responses are described below. For further detail the reader is referred to references 13 and 14.

PHYSIOLOGICAL ACTIONS

The physiological actions of glucagon are summarized in Table 2. Glucagon was initially thought to be of some importance in the homeostatic normalization of plasma glucose from hypoglycaemic levels. Recent investigations, however, have elucidated a central role of glucagon in the protection against hypoglycaemia. These investigations have indicated that glucagon is the primary defence against hypoglycaemia, with epinephrine having only a secondary role as a 'back-up' mechanism, and growth hormone, cortisol and neurally released norepinephrine providing no immediate contribution at all[15-18].

Another important action of glucagon is in the situation of ingestion of protein alone. Although not usually the case with food intake in man, such occurrences are not infrequent. In the carnivorous animal kingdom however this is a frequent occurrence. Due to aminogenic stimulation of insulin in the absence of carbohydrate intake hypoglycaemia would ensue were it not for the concomitant stimulation of glucagon by amino acids[19].

Exercise represents the prototype physiological stress situation calling for an integrated pattern of physiological adaptation. Among the requirements of the exercise state is a rapid availability of glucose to provide fuel for working muscle mass. Exercise induced glucagon stimulation promotes this action[20]. Other stress situations including fever, sepsis, fear and shock states, are accompanied by similar glucagon elevations, proportional to the degree of

Table 2   Physiological actions of glucagon

Protection against fasting hypoglycaemia	First defence
Protein meal	Prevents hypoglycaemia that would otherwise occur from insulin secretion
Exercise	Increases glucose availability by promoting hepatic glucose production
Stress	Increases glucose availability by promoting hepatic glucose production

such stress, which essentially subserve the same physiological role as exercise[21]. The above physiological actions are all therefore promoted by the physiological hyperglucagonaemia which accompanies them. With the exception of the special circumstance of protein ingestion however, these physiological responses occur in the face of reciprocal changes in plasma insulin levels. Accordingly the prevailing insulin:glucagon ratio is the important determinant of glucose disposal patterns at any given moment[22]. Elevated insulin levels can override or suppress many of these actions of glucagon. In exercise, despite insulin suppression necessary to promote fuel availability, a low level of insulin is necessary to enable glucose uptake by working muscle.

DISTURBANCES IN PLASMA LEVELS

The major disturbances in plasma glucagon levels are summarized in Table 3. Hyperglucagonaemia is most often seen in a few clinical situations but is also present in a number of uncommon circumstances. The common conditions of pathological hyperglucagonaemia are diabetes, where glucagon elevations are inversely related to degree of diabetic control[23-26], and shock states[21,27].

Table 3   Abnormalities of circulating glucagon

Hyperglucagonaemia	Hypoglucagonaemia

1. Diabetes
    Ketoacidosis
    Hyperosmolar syndrome
2. Chronic renal failure
3. Shock states:
        Myocardial infarction
        Septicaemia
        Burns
        Haemorrhagea
        Hypovolaemia
4. Acute pancreatitis
5. Cirrhosis
    Portaeaval shunting ⟨Natural / Surgical⟩
6. Glucagonoma
7. [Glucagon antibodies in
        insulin requiring diabetics]
8. Familial hyperglucagonaemia
    (asymptomatic)
	1. Infant of diabetic mother
	2. ?Isolated functional defect
	    of glucagon release
	3. Chronic pancreatitis
	    Pancreatectomy
	    Extensive pancreatic cancer
	    Cystic fibrosis

Hyperglucagonaemia is also present in acute pancreatitis[13], glucagonoma syndrome [13,28], a rare familial hyperglucagonaemia[29], chronic renal failure[30], cirrhosis and liver failure[31-33], and portacaval shunts[34]. In the latter cases the hyperglucagonaemia arises predominantly from reduced or absent metabolic disposal of glucagon by the kidney or liver, as discussed below. In all of these situations (other than the familial hyperglucagonaemia, which occurs in healthy individuals), pathological hyperglucagonaemia contributes to the metabolic disturbances associated with these clinical conditions. Hypoglucagonaemia is not a well described or common clinical entity although it is possible that isolated glucagon deficiency syndromes do exist. Thus, a few cases of glucagon deficiency have been reported in infants, children and adults[35,36]. Hypoglucagonaemia will, of course, also be present in situations of extensive disease of the pancreas, or pancreatectomy, although, due to concomitant insulin deficiency, its metabolic consequences are not striking. It may, however, be related to hypoglycaemic tendencies in such patients treated with insulin for their secondary diabetes. Finally, it has been suggested that due to prevailing hyperglycaemia *in utero*, the infant of the diabetic mother in addition to developing hyperinsulinaemia, also may have hypoglucagonaemia due to suppression of A-cell development. This dual defect has been postulated to be responsible for the profound, unresponsive hypoglycaemic episodes that such infants are prone to develop.

METABOLISM

As is the case for other hormones, an appreciation of glucagon metabolism in the body is important for the understanding of disturbances of the plasma glucagon levels and chromatographic profiles in various disease states. After the findings of hyperglucagonaemia in chronic renal failure, by Bilbrey and co-workers, shown to be correctable by transplantation but not by haemodialysis[30], initial studies into the metabolism of glucagon revealed that the kidney was an important site of metabolic disposal of the peptide[13,14]. With the demonstration of molecular heterogeneity in man, it became important to assess the role of the kidney in determining IRG. Kuku *et al.*[37] observed that the hyperglucagonaemia of renal failure was due largely to a striking elevation of the 9000 mol. wt. (B-peak) fraction, which comprised 56% of the total IRG level of 535 pg/ml. A moderate elevation of the C-peak fraction ($\approx 30\%$) also occurred. It was subsequently found[38] that the 3500 mol. wt., biologically active component is metabolized by both glomerular filtration and by the renal tubules after uptake from the peritubular blood, whereas the 9000 mol. wt. (B-peak) component is metabolized solely by the latter mechanism. Thus, only in nephrectomized rats, did this B-peak component appear and the appearance and progressive increase could be followed sequentially after bilateral nephrectomy in rats (Figure 3). These observations explain the hyperglucagonaemia and abnormal chromatographic profiles seen in uraemic subjects. Moreover, since only the 3500 mol. wt. component is biologically responsive, this also accounts for the disturbances in plasma glucagon response to oral glucose or intravenous arginine initially observed in uraemic patients[39]. This is illustrated in Figure 4. Thus, due to the large contribution of the 9000 mol. wt. (B-peak) component in uraemic

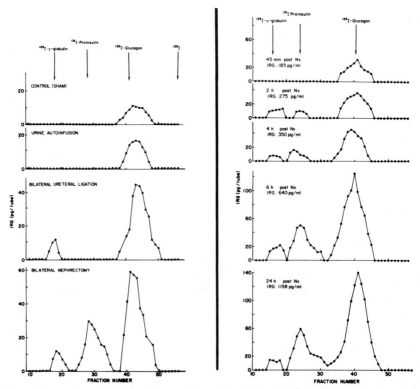

Figure 3 *Left:* Representative elution profiles of circulating IRG 24 h after surgery in a sham operated rat, a urine auto-infused rat, a rat with bilateral ureteral ligation, and a rat 24 h after bilateral nephrectomy. The ∼9000 mol. wt. fraction was found only in neprectomized rats.

Right: Representative plasma IRG elution profiles on 1 × 50 cm Biogel P-30 columns before and at various intervals after nephrectomy. Note the progressive increment in 3500 mol. wt. IRG (peak C) and in particular 9000 mol. wt. IRG (peak B) following renal ablation. Columns were calibrated with [^{125}I]-γ-globulin (mol. wt. >40 000), [^{131}I]-proinsulin (mol. wt. 9000) and [^{125}I]-glucagon (mol. wt. 3500) (Emmanouel, D. S. *et al.*, 1976. Reprinted, with permission, from *J. Clin. Invest.*, **58**, 1266)

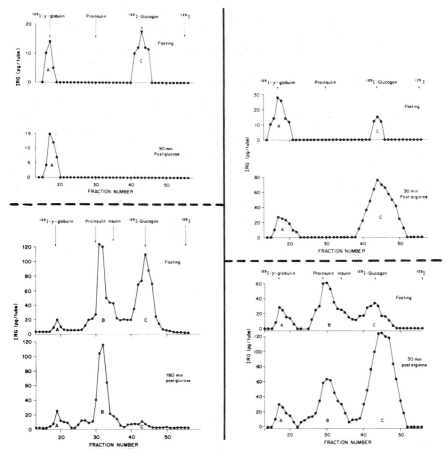

Figure 4 *Left*: Representative elution profiles of plasma IRG on 1 × 50 cm Biogel P-30 columns before and after 100 g oral glucose in a normal patient (above) and a patient with chronic renal failure (below).

Right: Representative elution profile of plasma IRG on similar columns before and after intravenous arginine infusion in a normal subject (above) and a patient with chronic renal failure (below). The arginine was infused over 30 min at a dose of 500 mg/kg in the healthy subject and 250 mg/kg in the CRF patient. Columns were calibrated with [^{125}I]-γ-globulin (mol. wt. > 40 000), proinsulin (9000 mol. wt.), insulin (6000 mol. wt.) and [^{125}I]-glucagon (3500 mol. wt.). (Kuku, S. F. *et al.*, 1976. Reprinted, with permission, from *J. Clin. Invest.*, **58**, 742)

plasma, which is not responsive to suppressive or stimulatory influences, oral glucose results in decreased suppressibility of whole plasma IRG and intravenous arginine, and in impaired stimulation of whole plasma IRG, despite quantitatively normal responses of the biologically active 3500 mol. wt. (C-peak) component in uraemic subjects.

Subsequent studies revealed that the liver also plays a major role in glucagon disposal[40]. It was shown that hepatic extraction of glucagon contributes about 35% to total metabolic clearance and renal extraction a similar amount (Figure 5). Thus, both organs contribute about one-third of the total metabolic clearance of glucagon. Of the remaining one-third, the bulk appears to be contributed by splanchnic metabolism[40]. However, in the case of the liver, unlike the kidney which metabolizes both 3500 mol. wt. and 9000 mol. wt. IRG components, predilection for 3500 mol. wt. IRG was demonstrated[41]. This was later confirmed by fully quantitating transhepatic balance of IRG components by means of hepatic blood flow measurements[42]. This predilection for 3500 mol. wt. IRG extraction by the liver is shown in Figure 6. In both normal and uraemic rats, only this component is diminished in traversing the liver. The same is true in dogs[41] and man[42].

These observations on hepatic extraction of glucagon have a number of important implications in the interpretation of the experimental data related to glucagon action at the liver, and for the understanding of glucagon

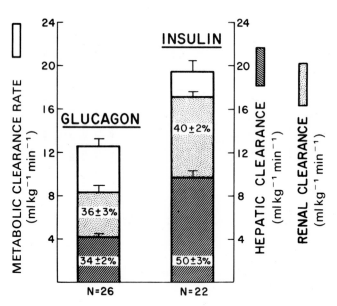

Figure 5 Simultaneously measured metabolic clearance rates and hepatic and renal clearance of exogenously infused glucagon and insulin in dogs. Contribution of hepatic and renal metabolism to total metabolic clearance for each hormone is shown within the hatched panel.

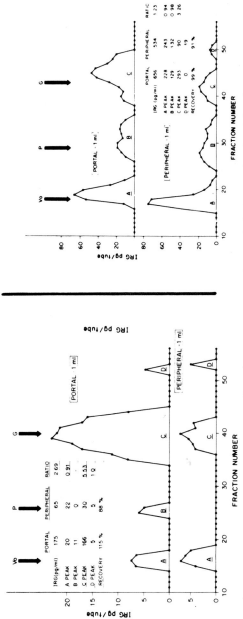

Figure 6 Gel filtration profiles of plasma IRG in simultaneously drawn portal and peripheral samples in a healthy rat (left panel) and a rat 24 h post-nephrectomy (right panel). Vo = void volume (mol. wt. >40000), P = proinsulin (mol. wt. = 9000) and G = glucagon (mol. wt. = 3500). Columns were calibrated as in Figure 5. (Jaspan, J. B. *et al.*, 1977. Reprinted, with permission, from *J. Clin. Invest.*, **60**, 421).

13

pathophysiology in general. In this light, peripheral glucagon estimations will lead to a serious under-estimation of the amount of glucagon to which the liver is exposed during the critical 'first pass' when most of its biological action is being exerted. In addition, during somatostatin suppression of glucagon secretion in the presence of hypoglycaemia, it has been noted that there is a glucagon 'breakthrough' of suppression. In one study, although peripheral glucagon levels were elevated (146 pg/ml), the degree of glucagon secretion during such suppression was under-estimated from peripheral glucagon levels, by a factor of 3, as simultaneously measured portal glucagon levels were 350 pg/ml[43]. Moreover, it has been noted that hepatic glucagon extraction varies widely from animal to animal[40]. Predictions of portal glucagon levels under any given set of physiological or pathological circumstances are further called into question, since it is probable that many factors, such as the rate of secretion, nutritional status, food intake and disease states, may influence glucagon extraction. Thus, studies that attempt to interpret the physiological actions of glucagon and its role in disease based upon peripheral hormone concentrations alone may be inaccurate.

ROLE OF GLUCAGON DISTURBANCES IN DISEASE

Disturbances in glucagon secretion and metabolism in a variety of diseases, and the resultant hyperglucagonaemia, may contribute significantly to, or even account for, the metabolic disturbances characteristic of these conditions.

(a) Diabetes

Hyperglucagonaemia in diabetes is well recognized[23-26]. The elevated glucagon levels are due to hypersecretion, although the possible contribution of decreased metabolic clearance by liver and/or kidney has not been excluded. The hyperglucagonaemia of diabetes is due largely to elevation of the biologically active 3500 mol. wt. fraction[13]. As mentioned previously, the degree of hyperglucagonaemia is related to the level of blood sugar control, tending to be greatest in more severely hyperglycaemic diabetics and particularly so in ketoacidosis and hyperosmolar syndrome[44]. The prevailing degree of hyperglucagonaemia in turn contributes to the hyperglycaemia in these insulin deficient states and is also of fundamental importance in producing accelerated ketosis both by virtue of accelerated lipolysis and promotion of hepatic ketogenesis by activation of the hepatic carnitine acyl transferase enzyme system[45].

(b) Chronic renal failure

The hyperglucagonaemia of renal failure discussed in more detail above is due to elevations in both 3500 mol. wt. (biologically active) and 9000 mol. wt. (biologically inactive) components (see Figure 4), the latter being dominant. Carbohydrate intolerance, which is characteristic of uraemia, appears to be due to enhanced sensitivity of the liver to glucagon and impaired sensitivity of insulin sensitive tissues to insulin, with insulin resistance[46], rather than the disturbances in the levels of these hormones *per se.*

(c) Glucagonoma

The glucagonoma syndrome[13,28] due to A-cell tumours of the pancreas (usually malignant) is accompanied by markedly elevated plasma glucagon levels. The clinical features of the syndrome are summarized in Table 4. The non-ketotic hyperglycaemia, hypoaminoacidaemia, weight loss and proximal muscle weakness are directly attributable to the hyperglycaemic and catabolic actions of glucagon. Although less clearly established, the characteristic skin rash and mucous membrane disorder, anaemia, and neurologic deficit (described in a few cases), are probably also attributable to the grossly elevated plasma glucagon levels. The diagnosis of glucagonoma is usually made clinically in the presence of many of the features shown in Table 4. The skin rash is highly suggestive of such a diagnosis clinically and is pathognomonic histopathologically consisting of necrosis and bullae in the upper epidermal layers. However, the skin rash is absent in about one-third to one-quarter of patients[28]. In such circumstances chromatographic analysis of plasma is diagnostic. This procedure also provides important confirmation or exclusion of the diagnosis in questionable cases. Plasma glucagon levels are usually very high but, especially when they are not inordinately raised, this may be

Table 4   Glucagonoma syndrome

Necrolytic migratory erythema
Stomatitis/glossitis
Anaemia
Weight loss
Diabetes
Hyperglucagonaemia
Hypoaminoacidaemia
(? neurological deficit)

The above clinical picture occurs in association with α-cell tumour of pancreatic islets

attributable to other conditions (for example, diabetes, renal failure or liver disease). However, on chromatography, the diagnostic feature is the presence of large amounts of the 9000 mol. wt. component, believed to be a product peptide of proglucagon. This finding is analogous to the presence of elevated proinsulin levels in insulinoma and of other prohormones in certain endocrine tumours. This is illustrated in Figure 7, which shows the chromatographic profiles in five proven cases of glucagonoma, all showing striking elevations of the 9000 mol. wt., B-peak fraction. The only other condition in which this occurs is chronic renal failure, which can easily be distinguished on clinical grounds.

(d) Hepatic failure; porto-systemic shunting

Glucagon levels are also elevated in liver disease, liver failure, and porto-systemic shunting without significant liver disease[31-34]. The carbohydrate intolerance noted in these conditions has been linked to these disturbances of glucagon, although it is difficult to ascertain whether this is a primary or causative factor, or part of a more generalized metabolic disturbance related to impaired hepatocyte function and glucagon and insulin metabolism. An important consideration in this regard is the diversion of glucagon and insulin past the liver with shunting which frequently accompanies severe liver disease of a cirrhotic nature. In this regard it has been suggested[32] that a normal negative feedback signal from the liver (perhaps a metabolic intermediate resulting from the action of glucagon at the liver) to the A-cells of the pancreas is interrupted, resulting in glucagon hypersecretion. Increased sensitivity of

---

Figure 7 Elution patterns of plasma immunoreactive glucagon on 1 × 50 cm Biogel P-30 columns in five patients with glucagonoma. Column calibrations were as in Figure 6. Additional clinical details in these patients are as follows: Panel 1: 53 years, female, diabetic 10 years, initially treated with tolbutamide and subsequently with insulin, up to 35 U per day, with poor control; large malignant glucagonoma in pancreas with extensive hepatic and peritoneal metastases. Panel 2: 39 years, male, four-year history of necrolytic skin rash and weight loss; hypoaminoacidaemia; diabetic glucose tolerance curve; 4 × 4 cm glucagonoma in tail of pancreas with invasive characteristics but no metastases. Panel 3: 40 years, male, two-year history of weight loss, seven-month history of necrolytic skin rash; stomatitis, anaemia, hypoaminoacidaemia and diabetic glucose tolerance test; glucagonoma in body of pancreas and multiple hepatic metastases. Panel 4: 62 years, female, five-year history of diabetes, poorly controlled on insulin, with recurrent episodes of nonketotic hyperglycaemia requiring hospitalization, and eventually leading to death. Specimen taken six hours postmortem: 0.4 cm glucagonoma in body of pancreas with invasive characteristics but no metastases. Panel 5: 37 years, male, 1½-year history of skin rash, weight loss, diabetes, hypoaminoacidaemia, and metabolic encephalopathy; malignant glucagonoma with hepatic metastases. (Jaspan, J. B. and Rubenstein, A. H., 1977. Reprinted, with permission, from *Diabetes*, **26**, 887)

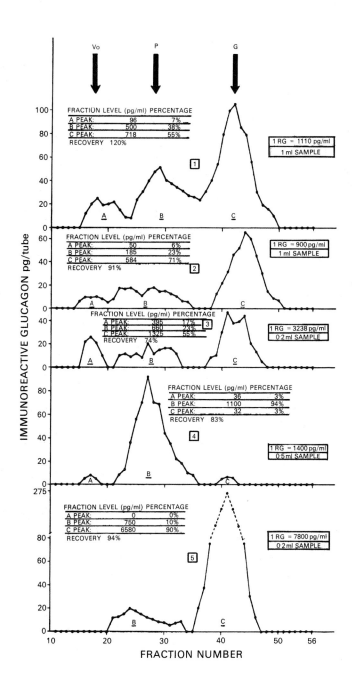

the liver to glucagon has also been proposed as a factor in the abnormal carbohydrate tolerance of liver disease. Hepatic encephalopathy has also been attributed to hyperglucagonaemia characteristic of shunting, possibly related to the rampant protein catabolism which is associated with the hyperglucagonaemia[34]. The encephalopathy of the glucagonoma syndrome[13] may have a similar basis.

(e) Post-pancreatectomy; isolated glucagon deficiency

Although in animals absence of the pancreas is not associated with glucagon deficiency because of glucagon secretion, which may actually be increased, from A-cells in stomach and upper small bowel[9,47], pancreatectomy in man is usually associated with glucagon deficiency. The metabolic consequences of glucagon deficiency in pancreatectomy diabetes are, if anything, beneficial, since in contrast to spontaneously occurring diabetes where hyperglucagonaemia aggravates carbohydrate intolerance[44], glucagon deficiency appears to render such diabetic patients more stable and easier to control. On the other hand, in the absence of glucagon, these patients are often more susceptible to insulin induced hypoglycaemia. Moreover, although glucagon is a primary factor in promoting ketogenesis[45], particularly in the insulin deficient state, development of ketosis has been shown to be possible in pancreatomized man[48]. Finally, sporadic cases of isolated glucagon deficiency with resultant hypoglycaemia have been reported[35,36].

SUMMARY AND OVERVIEW

Over the 60 years since its recognition, glucagon has risen from the status of another pancreatic peptide, to the point where today, this hormone is recognized as a key factor in intermediary metabolism, contributing in a major way to the maintenance of normal metabolism during ambient and stress states and to the metabolic disturbances of a wide variety of clinical diseases. In addition, a number of entirely unrelated and somewhat surprising pharmacologic actions have come to the fore, with important clinical or potential clinical applications. These include a cardiotropic action, an hepatic and intestinal regenerative capacity, and actions on intestinal, biliary and portal vein smooth musculature, on gastric acid secretion and bile flow. A complete understanding of the role of glucagon in health and disease, as well as an appreciation of therapeutic usefulness and limitations, necessitates knowledge of patterns and controls of secretion, molecular heterogeneity, variable sensitivity of target tissues, and normal and deranged metabolic disposal of this interesting peptide.

References

1. Banting, F. G. and Best, C. H. (1922). The internal secretion of the pancreas. *J. Lab. Clin. Med.*, **7**, 251
2. Kimball, C. P. and Murlin, J. R. (1924). Aqueous extracts of pancreas. III. Some precipitation reactions of insulin. *J. Biol. Chem.*, **58**, 337
3. Sundby, F. (1974). Species variation in the primary structure of glucagon. *Metabolism*, **25** (Suppl. 1), 1319
4. Wunsch, F. and Weinges, K. F. (1972). The synthesis of glucagon. Properties of synthetic glucagon. In Lefèbvre, P. J. and Unger, R. H. (eds.) *Glucagon: Molecular Physiology, Clinical and Therapeutic Implications*, pp. 31–46. (Oxford: Pergamon)
5. Steiner, D. F., Cunningham, D. D., Spigelman, L. and Atten, B. (1967). Insulin biosynthesis: Evidence for a precursor. *Science*, **157**, 699
6. Tager, H. S. (1981). Biosynthesis of glucagon. In Unger, R. H. and Orci, L. (eds.) *Glucagon*, pp. 39–54. (New York: Elsevier North Holland)
7. Koranyi, L., Peterfy, F., Szabo, J., Torok, A., Guoth, M. and Tamas, G. (1981). Evidence for transformation of glucagon-like immunoreactivity of gut into pancreatic glucagon in vivo., *Diabetes*, **30**, 792
8. Orci, L. and Perrelet, A. (1981). The morphology of the A-cell. In Unger, R. H. and Orci, L. (eds.) *Glucagon*, pp. 3–36. (New York: Elsevier North Holland)
9. Conlon, J. M. (1981). Molecular forms of the glucagon-like polypeptides (IRG and GLI) in tissues and plasma. In Unger, R. H. and Orci, L. (eds.) *Glucagon*, pp. 55–75. (New York: Elsevier North Holland)
10. Boden, G. (1981). Extrapancreatic glucagon in human subjects. In Unger, R. H. and Orci, L. (eds.) *Glucagon*, pp. 349–357. (New York: Elsevier North Holland)
11. Unger, R. H., Dobbs, R. and Orci. L. (1978). Insulin, glucagon and somatostatin secretion in the regulation of metabolism. *Ann. Rev. Physiol.*, **200**, 307
12. Leclercq-Meyer, V., Rebolleto, O., Marchand, J. and Malaisse, W. J. (1975). Glucagon release: Paradoxical stimulation of glucagon during calcium deprivation. *Science*, **189**, 897
13. Jaspan, J. B. and Rubenstein, A. H. (1977). Circulating glucagon: Plasma profiles and metabolism in health and disease. *Diabetes*, **26**, 887
14. Jaspan, J. B., Polonsky, K. S. and Rubenstein, A. H. (1981). The heterogeneity of immunoreactive glucagon in plasma: Clinical implications. In Unger, R. H. and Orci, L. (eds.) *Glucagon*, pp. 77–96. (New York: Elsevier North Holland)
15. Cherrington, A. D. and Liljenquist, J. E. (1981). Role of glucagon in regulating glucose production in vivo. In Unger, R. H. and Orci, L. (eds.) *Glucagon*, pp. 221–253. (New York: Elsevier North Holland)
16. Rizza, R., Cryer, P. and Gerich, J. (1979). Role of glucagon, catecholamines and growth hormone in human glucose counter regulation. *J. Clin. Invest.*, **64**, 62
17. Gerich, J., Davis, J., Lorenzi, M., Rizza, R., Bohannon, N., Karam, J., Lewis, S., Kaplan, R., Schultz, T. and Cryer, P. (1979). Hormonal mechanisms of recovery from insulin induced hypoglycemia in man. *Am. J. Physiol.*, **236**, E380
18. Santiago, J., Clarke, W., Shah, S. and Cryer, P. (1980). Epinephrine, norepinephrine, glucagon and growth hormone released in association with physiological decrements in the plasma glucose concentration in normal and diabetic man. *J. Clin. Endocrinol. Metab.*, **51**, 877

19. Aguilar-Parada, E., Eisentraut, A. N. and Unger, R. (1969). Effects of starvation on pancreatic glucagon secretion in man. *Diabetes*, **18**, 717

20. Kemmer, F. and Vranic, M. (1981). The role of glucagon and its relationship to other glucoregulatory hormones in exercise. In Unger, R. H. and Orci, L. (eds.) *Glucagon*, pp. 297–331. (New York: Elsevier North Holland)

21. Editorial (1975). Glucagon and shock. *J. Am. Med. Assoc.*, **233**, 1195

22. Unger, R. H. (1972). Insulin:glucagon ratio. *Isr. J. Med. Sci.*, **8**, 252

23. Unger, R. H. (1971). Glucagon physiology and pathophysiology. *N. Engl. J. Med.*, **285**, 443

24. Unger, R. H. and Orci, L. (1977). The role of glucagon in diabetes. *Arch. Intern. Med.*, **137**, 482

25. Unger, R. H. (1976), Glucagon and the insulin:glucagon ratio in diabetes and other catabolic illnesses. *Diabetes*, **20**, 834

26. Gerich, J. E. (1976). Alpha cell dysfunction in diabetes mellitus. *Metabolism*, **25** (Suppl. 1), 1513

27. Willerson, J., Hutcheson, D., Leshin, S., Faloona, G. and Unger, R. H. (1974). Serum glucagon and insulin levels and their relationship to blood glucose values in patients with acute myocardial infarction and acute coronary insufficiency. *Am. J. Med.*, **57**, 747

28. Bhathena, S., Higgins, G. and Recant, L. (1981). Glucagonoma and glucagonoma syndrome. In Unger, R. H. and Orci, L. (eds.) *Glucagon*, pp. 413–438. (New York: Elsevier North Holland)

29. Boden, G. and Owen, D. (1977). Familial hyperglucagonemia – an autosomal dominant disorder. *N. Engl. J. Med.*, **286**, 534

30. Bilbrey, G. L., Faloona, G. R., White, M. G., Atkins, C., Hull, A. R. and Knochel, I. P. (1975). Hyperglucagonemia in uremia: Reversal by renal transplantation. *Ann. Intern. Med.*, **82**, 525

31. Marco, J., Diego, J., Villanueva, M., Diaz-Ferros, M., Valverde, I. and Segovia, J. (1973). Elevated glucagon levels in cirrhosis of the liver. *N. Engl. J. Med.*, **289**, 1197

32. Sherwin, R., Fisher, M., Bessoff, J., Snyder, M., Hendler, R., Conn, H. and Felig, P. (1978). Hyperglucagonemia in cirrhosis: Altered secretion and sensitivity to glucagon. *Gastroenterology*, **74**, 1224

33. Sherwin, R., Joshi, P., Hendler, R., Felig, P. and Conn, H. (1974). Hyperglucagonemia in Laennec's cirrhosis. *N. Engl. J. Med.*, **290**, 239

34. Soeters, P., Weir, G., Ebeid, A. M., James, J. H. and Fischer, J. E. (1975). Insulin and glucagon following porto-caval shunt. *Gastroenterology*, **69**, A-67, 867 (Abstr.)

35. Vidness, J. and Oyasaeter, S. (1977). Glucagon deficiency causing severe neonatal hypoglycemia in a patient with normal insulin secretion. *Ped. Res.*, **11**, 943

36. Grollman. A., McCaleb, W. and White, F. (1964). Glucagon deficiency as cause of hypoglycemia. *Metabolism*, **13**, 686

37. Kuku, S. F., Jaspan, J. B., Emmanouel, D., Zeidler, A., Katz, A. I. and Rubenstein, A. H. (1976). Heterogeneity of plasma glucagon: Circulating components in normal subjects and patients with chronic renal failure. *J. Clin. Invest.*, **58**, 742

38. Emmanouel, D. S., Jaspan, J. B., Kuku, S. F., Rubenstein, A. H. and Katz, I. (1976). Pathogenesis and characterization of hyperglucagonemia in the uremic rat. *J. Clin. Invest.*, **58**, 1266

39. Bilbrey, G., Faloona, G., White, M. and Knochel, J. P. (1974). Hyperglucagonemia of renal failure. *J. Clin. Invest.*, **53**, 841

40. Jaspan, J. B., Polonsky, K. S., Lewis, M., Pensler, J., Pugh, W., Moossa, A. and Rubenstein, A. H. (1981). Hepatic metabolism of glucagon in the dog. Contribution of the liver to the overall metabolic disposal of glucagon. *Am. J. Physiol.*, **240**, E233

41. Jaspan, J. B., Huen, A., Morley, C., Moossa, A. and Rubenstein, A. H. (1977). The role of the liver in glucagon metabolism. *J. Clin. Invest.*, **60**, 421

42. Jaspan, J. B., Polonsky, K. S., Röjdmark, S., Ishida, T., Field, J., and Rubenstein, A. (1981). Hepatic extraction of plasma immunoreactive glucagon components. Predilction for 3500 Dalton glucagon metabolism by the liver. *Diabetes*, **30**, 767

43. Polonsky, K. S., Jaspan, J. B., Pugh, W., Dhorajiwala, J., Abraham, M., Blix, P. and Moossa, A. (1981). Insulin and glucagon breakthrough of somatostatin suppression. Importance of portal vein hormone measurements. *Diabetes*, **30**, 664

44. Gerich, J. (1977). On the causes and consequences of abnormal glucagon secretion in human diabetes mellitus. In Foa, P., Bajaj, J. and Foa, N. (eds.) *Glucagon: Its Role in Physiology and Clinical Medicine*, pp. 607–615. (New York: Springer)

45. McGarry, J. D. and Foster, D. W. (1981). Ketogenesis. In Unger, R. H. and Orci, L. (eds.) *Glucagon*, pp. 273–295. (New York: Elsevier North Holland)

46. Sherwin, R. S., Bastl, C., Finkelstein, F. O., Fischer, M., Black, H., Hendler, R. and Felig. P. (1976). Influence of uremia and hemodialysis on the turnover and metabolic effects of glucagon. *J. Clin. Invest.*, **57**, 722

47. Lefèbvre, P. and Luyckx, A. S. (1981). Extra pancreatic glucagon. In Unger, R. H. and Orci, L. (eds.) *Glucagon*, pp. 335–348. (New York: Elsevier North Holland)

48. Barnes, A. J., Bloom, S. R. and Alberti, K. G. (1977). Ketoacidosis in pancreatectomized man. *N. Engl. J. Med.*, **296**, 1250

Address for correspondence

Dr. J. B. Jaspan,
Department of Medicine,
University of Chicago,
950 East 59th Street,
Chicago, IL 60637, USA

DISCUSSION

Oriol Bosch: Does the fact that the B-peak does not decrease through the liver passage mean that there is no binding and, therefore, no liver action, or is just not detectable by present methods?

Jaspan: This is an important point. We believe that there is no binding and therefore it is not recognized and not degraded. Some 7–8 years ago, Terris and Steiner, from the University of Chicago, suggested that degradation of peptides by the liver was not regulated independently of their binding, as was previously believed to be the case. They showed a relationship between binding and degradation of insulin *in vitro*, and although this was initially challenged, most subsequent work has tended to confirm this (Terris, S. and Steiner, D. (1975). *J. Biol. Chem.*, **250**, 8389; (1976). *J. Clin. Invest.*, **57**, 885). We believe that what happens with respect to glucagon is that the C-peak (biologically active component) is recognized and that once receptor binding takes place, both action and degradation are initiated and can be paralleled. Our recent studies with dogs *in vivo* have shown this to be so. We fed dogs glucose and what happened was that the insulin extraction went up from the basal of 30% to about 60%; in other words, there was an absolute increase in hepatic insulin extraction at the same time as the liver started taking up glucose, and we could correlate the hepatic glucose uptake which, of course, is a measure of the biological activity of insulin, with the degradation. I think it likely that a number of peptide hormones are degraded in proportion to their action. Slatopolsky and Klahr and their colleagues in studies with parathyroid hormone metabolism found that parathyroid hormone, which is rather actively degraded by the liver, also, for reasons that are not yet clear, increases hepatic glucose output (Martin, K. *et al.* (1976). *J. Clin. Invest.*, **58**, 781). When these authors then made a carboxyl terminus tryptic digest of parathyroid hormone they found it had no effect on glucose metabolism by the liver and also that it was not degraded by liver (Hruska, K. *et al.* (1979). *J. Clin. Invest.*, **64**, 1016).

Diamant: How do you think it is related to glicetin?

Jaspan: Studies have suggested that proglucagon is an 18 000 dalton peptide, and what I termed the B-peak is a stable intermediate cleavage form. There are probably a series of intermediate cleavages, some of which are labile. Thus this B-peak fraction found in plasma is probably not the proglucagon gene sequence product but rather an intermediate cleavage form that is stable, which accounts for it being found in plasma. It has been called 'proglucagon', though in the strictest sense of the word this is probably not correct.

Diamant: How do you think it is related to glicentin?

Jaspan: They are related peptides. In all probability they are derived from a common gene product, with differential post-synthetic modification in gut and pancreas subsequently resulting in the structural differences of the two peptides. Thus glicentin (molecular weight ≈ 12 000) includes the 29 amino acid sequence of glucagon, with an approximately 60 amino acid amino terminus extension and 8 amino acid carboxyl terminus extension. Proglucagon, the primary gene product (molecular weight 18 000), is extended an extra 50 amino acids at the amino terminus, and is probably identical at the carboxyl terminus. Glicentin is therefore formed from the gene product by cleavage of this ≈ 6000 dalton amino terminus. The B-peak (molecular weight ≈ 9000–12 000) in plasma in renal failure, in glucagonoma patients, and in smaller amounts in normal dogs, represents a similar although slightly more extensive cleavage at the amino terminus, but cleavage of the entire carboxyl terminus extension does yield the free carboxyl terminus present in glucagon itself. For this reason, antisera which react with the central portion of the glucagon molecule, so-called non-specific antisera, will react with glicentin, proglucagon, the 9000 dalton of intermediate cleavage product of proglucagon (B-peak), and glucagon itself. On the other hand, an immunogenic determinant in the structure of glucagon that is not present in glicentin nor in other C-terminally extended forms, appears to reside in the free C-terminus of glucagon or in the carboxyl terminal segment of the peptide. Thus, antibodies which are raised against the 11 amino acid C-terminal tryptic digest of glucagon or carboxyl terminus, specific antibodies like 30-K, do not react with glicentin or other C- or N-terminus extensions and are, therefore, termed 'glucagon specific'. This is described in more detail in the Tager reference I have cited in my paper (Tager, H. S. (1981). In Unger, R. H. and Orci, L. (eds.) *Glucagon*, pp. 77–96 (New York: Elsevier North Holland).

Diamant: Firstly, the primary structure of porcine glicentin was recently determined to consist of 69 amino acids (Thim, L. and Moody, A. J. (1981). *Regulatory Peptides*, **2**, 239). They found that the amino acid extension of glucagon contains 30 and not 60 amino acids and was denoted GRPP (glicentin related pancreatic peptide). The three sequences of glicentin (GRPP, glucagon hexapeptide) are linked by two LYS-ARG pairs which probably represent the sites for post-synthetic enzymatic cleavages. Secondly, I wonder if in the renal failure situation this B-peak might possibly originate from gut glucagon-like material and not predominantly from the pancreas.

Jaspan: I would agree with what you say. As I mentioned, both glicentin in gut and glucagon in pancreas come from the same gene product. The reason that you find different proportions in different tissues is because the processing, presumably due to different enzyme systems, is different in the two tissues. Glicentin can theoretically be cleaved to a fragment that is the B-peak. The 9000 dalton component in plasma arises in pancreas because bowel appears to lack the enzymes that effect carboxyl cleavage. Of course in animals bowel has A-cells, so I should say that it is an A-cell product rather than a bowel product. Thus in dogs and other animals you will find this material in gut, where it is in A-cells, in stomach, and upper small bowel. If you look at small bowel glucagon immunoreactivity with specific carboxyl terminus directed antibodies you will not detect any glicentin. However, large amounts of glicentin are detectable with centrally directed (specific) antibodies. The same is true in plasma, and it is for this reason that assessment of glucagon physiology and levels must depend on carboxyl terminus specific (non-cross reacting) antibodies.

Skucas: It has been found empirically that patients with chronic renal failure and diabetes do not react in the same way as normal patients to an intravenous dose of glucagon. They do not achieve the same degree of hypotonia. I was wondering if this effect in these patients may be due to the elevated glucagon levels.

Jaspan: Yes, I think that entirely possible. I am not aware of that literature to know exactly how it has been studied, but certainly the elevated glucagon levels that are present in renal failure (both the biological inactive peak which is just a function of metabolism, and also the truly active peak) could down regulate receptors. It is well known now that insulin and other hormones, including in this case glucagon, by virtue of the chronic hyperglucagonaemia, could well down regulate receptors so that response to a bolus would be sub-maximal. This is certainly conceivable. In fact studies by Sherwin, at Yale, have shown that sensitivity to glucagon rather than the disturbed levels of the hormone is what is altered in renal failure.

Christiansen: I should like to make a comment concerning the occurrence of glucagon in the human stomach. Recently studies by Dr. Jens Holst of our group in Copenhagen have shown virtually no glucagon in any part of the stomach, whereas somatostatin was found not only in the antrum, but also in the fundic region (unpublished data).

Jaspan: Is that when you have looked at it immunohistochemically?

Christiansen: Yes.

Jaspan: That has been reported by other workers too. Many people have tried very hard to find glucagon in the gut of man. Boden has published some data suggesting that there may be some glucagon; others have done total pancreatectomies, shown that they were total by looking at insulin or C peptides levels, which were zero so there was no question that the pancreas was gone, and still detected glucagon. My explanation though, is that if you detect what looks like glucagon in an immunoassay, there are many things that cross-react, and so immunoreactivity with an antibody should not be taken as equal to glucagon, and I would not be surprised if in fact man has eliminated glucagon from gut, whereas more primitive animal species have retained it.

Diamant: In relation to that point, were the antibodies used in the study directed to the C-terminal or to the central portion of glucagon?

Christiansen: I am not an immunologist so I hesitate to answer, but I think it was the C-terminal.

Jaspan: Yes, I would concur with that. If an N-terminal antibody is used, one will pick up all the other non-glucagon peptides of gut, so I think one would almost certainly have to use an antibody directed towards the carboxyl end of the molecule which is specific for glucagon itself.

2

Structure-activity relationship for the spasmolytic action of glucagon

B. DIAMANT, K. D. JØRGENSEN and J. U. WEIS

STRUCTURE–ACTIVITY RELATIONSHIP (SAR) STUDIES ON METABOLIC EFFECTS OF GLUCAGON PEPTIDES

The entire glucagon molecule (Figure 1) is generally considered to be required in order that the full biological activity of this hormone be exerted, and cyclic AMP is believed to play a central role as a regulator of the effects elicited[1-4]. This concept has been well corroborated by SAR studies – of glucagon analogues and fragments. Studies in this area have focused mainly on evaluations of the various metabolic actions of glucagon, e.g., on its lipolytic and hyperglycaemic effects, as well as on its binding to liver cell membranes and on its activation of adenylate cyclase.

Grande et al. found that carbamylation of the N-terminal histidine markedly decreased the hyperglycaemic as well as the hyperlipaemic effects of glucagon in the duck[5]. Furthermore, glucagon-(2–29)-peptide was found by Lin et al. to be only a partial glucagon agonist, with a binding potency about 7% and an adenylate cyclase stimulating activity only 2% that of glucagon[6]. Similarly, Rodbell et al. found that removal of six of the C-terminal amino acids of glucagon resulted in an extensive loss both of binding and of adenylate

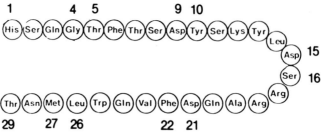

Figure 1   Amino acid sequence of native glucagon

cyclase activation[7]. Fragments of glucagon, such as glucagon-(1–21)-peptide, were found by Wright *et al.* to possess only 0.1 % of the potency of native glucagon as regards stimulation of cyclic AMP production and as regards binding to the glucagon receptor on liver cell membranes[8]. As pointed out by Frandsen *et al.*[9], the effects observed could be ascribed to contamination of the glucagon-(1–21)-peptide preparation by other biologically active glucagon analogues, such as glucagon methionine sulphoxide. The studies cited implicate the significance of the N-terminal and of the C-terminal part of the glucagon molecule for a full agonist effect.

Assan and Slusher[10] concluded from their studies with synthetic glucagon fragments in man that the lipolytic action of glucagon was contained within the (19–22) amino acid sequence, and the insulin-releasing and glycogenolytic actions within the (24–29) amino acids. In a recent study, Frandsen *et al.*[9] characterized several synthetic glucagon analogues in regard to receptor binding to purified rat liver plasma membranes, activation of adenylate cyclase in rat liver plasma membranes, and stimulation of lipolysis in isolated free fat cells from rat epididymal fat pad, and came to a somewhat different conclusion. As shown in Table 1, they found only glucagon-(5–29)-, glucagon-(1–4)–(10–29)-, and glucagon-(1–26)-peptides to have any affinity for the glucagon receptor in liver plasma membranes. The only analogue to exert any appreciable lipolytic or adenylcyclase activating effects was glucagon-(1–26)-peptide, but its potency in this respect was about 500 times less than that of native porcine glucagon. The obvious conclusion from the investigation of Frandsen *et al.*[9] is that the (27–29) amino acid sequence of glucagon is essential also for the lipolytic action of this hormone.

SAR STUDIES ON SPASMOLYTIC EFFECTS OF GLUCAGON PEPTIDES

Literature on SAR and the spasmolytic action of glucagon is relatively sparse. The generally accepted concept that the entire

Table 1   The effect of synthetic glucagon peptides on receptor binding, adenylcyclase activation, and lipolysis

Preparation	Receptor binding (in %)	Adenylcyclase activation (in %)	Lipolysis (in %)
Native porcine glucagon	100	100	100
Synthetic glucagon	108	—	—
Glucagon-(5–29)-peptide	5.7	<0.001	<0.01
Glucagon-(1–4)–(10–29)-peptide	0.47	<0.001	<0.01
Glucagon-(1–9)–(16–29)-peptide	0.0028	<0.001	<0.01
Glucagon-(1–15)–(22–29)-peptide	0.0017	<0.001	<0.01
Glucagon-(1–21)–(27–29)-peptide	0.0006	<0.001	<0.01
Glucagon-(1–26)-peptide	0.92	0.16	0.20

Data compiled from results given by Frandsen et al.[9]

glucagon molecule is needed for full biological activity is supported by Gagnon et al.[4] who found that glucagon-(2–29)-peptide possessed only 11 % of the spasmolytic activity of native glucagon, and that glucagon-(1–26)-peptide was completely inactive at concentrations nearly 40 times higher than the minimum effective dose of glucagon. It is important to emphasize that the experimental model used for these studies was the isolated rabbit renal artery contracted with noradrenalin.

In view of these results, we were surprised to find that the glucagon-(1–21)–(27–29)-peptide and the glucagon-(1–26)-peptide used in the study of Frandsen et al.[9] were equipotent with native glucagon in inhibiting the amplitude of contractions of the isolated guinea-pig ileum elicited by submaximal electrical stimulation (2 V, 0.2 pps, 50 ms) (Table 2). Furthermore, we found that glucagon-(1–21)-peptide obtained either by

Table 2   Relative molar potency of native glucagon and synthetic glucagon peptides on the inhibition of electrically stimulated guinea-pig ileum in vitro

Substance	Relative potency
Native glucagon	100
Glucagon-(1–26)-peptide	100
Glucagon-(1–21)–(27–29)-peptide	100
Glucagon-(1–21)-peptide	100
Glucagon-(1–20)-peptide	2
Glucagon-(1–19)-peptide	<0.03
Glucagon-(1–18)-peptide	<0.03
Glucagon-(2–21)-peptide	1

synthesis or by degradation of native glucagon followed by purification, was also equipotent with native glucagon as far as the spasmolytic action was concerned, both *in vitro* (electrically stimulated guinea-pig ileum (Figure 2) and rabbit gall bladder strips submaximally contracted with CCK-octapeptide (Figure 3)) and *in vivo* (motility inhibition registered by balloon catheters in rabbit duodenum, jejunum or colon (Figure 4), and enhancement of bile flow in rabbits (Figure 5) and rats (not shown)).

The potency of the spasmolytic action of synthetic glucagon-(2–21)-peptide was found to be about 1% of that of glucagon-(1–21)-peptide. The comparable value for glucagon-(1–20)-peptide was 2%, and for glucagon-(1–19)- and glucagon-(1–18)-peptides less than 0.03% (Table 2). This shows that the glucagon-(1–21)-peptide is the smallest fragment of glucagon to exert full spasmolytic activity, at least in the electrically stimulated guinea-pig ileum model.

We have also confirmed the spasmolytic action of glucagon on rabbit renal artery submaximally contracted with noradrenalin, as originally described by Gagnon et al.[3,4] With this preparation, glucagon-(1–21)-peptide was inactive at concentrations 100 times greater than those at which glucagon was active.

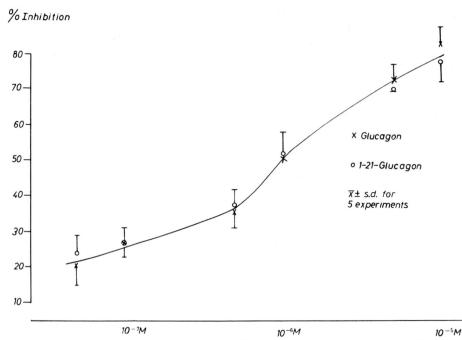

Figure 2   Dose–response relationship for the inhibitory action of glucagon and glucagon-(1–21)-peptide on the electrically stimulated guinea-pig ileum *in vitro*

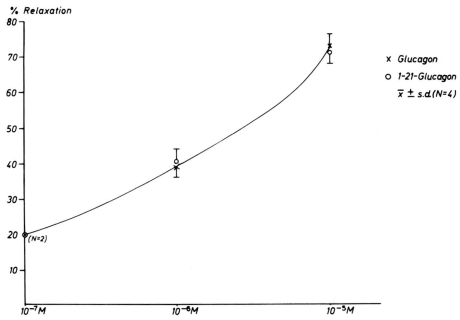

Figure 3 Dose–response relationship for the inhibitory action of glucagon and glucagon-(1–21)-peptide on rabbit gall bladder strips submaximally contracted with CCK-8 (0.1 µg/ml)

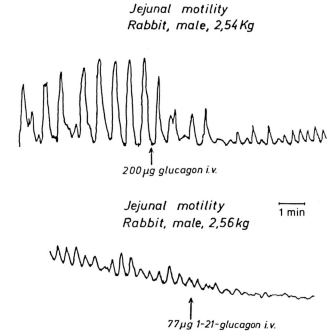

Figure 4 Motility inhibition of the rabbit jejunum *in vivo* induced by glucagon and glucagon-(1–21)-peptide, as registered by a balloon catheter

29

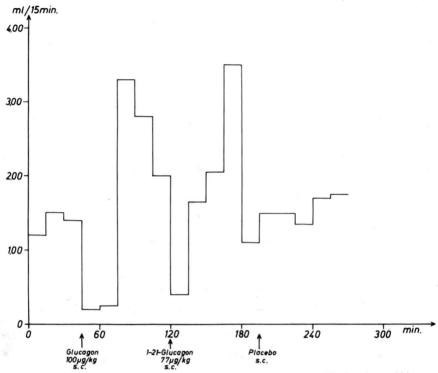

Figure 5 Influence of glucagon and glucagon-(1–21)-peptide on the bile flow in a rabbit, as registered by the use of a catheter in the bile duct

Furthermore, glucagon-(1–21)-peptide was not found to have an antagonistic effect against glucagon. Thus glucagon $(5 \times 10^{-7} \, \text{mol/l})$ inhibited the contractions induced by noradrenalin by 73% and this inhibition was not affected by the simultaneous presence of glucagon-(1–21)-peptide at concentrations which were five times higher. Noradrenalin-induced contractions of the rabbit renal artery can be decreased by a phosphodi-esterase inhibitor, such as theophylline. The spasmolytic action of glucagon is potentiated by theophylline in the model[3]. We have tried to demonstrate a latent inhibitory action of glucagon-(1–21)-peptide in the presence of theophylline, but without success.

The sensitivity of the rabbit portal vein to native glucagon is notably lower than that of the renal artery. Thus 300 times higher concentrations of glucagon were required to inhibit noradrenalin-induced contractions on the renal artery as compared to the portal vein. So far, we have not been able to demonstrate any inhibitory action of glucagon-(1–21)-peptide in this preparation.

30

POSSIBLE MECHANISM FOR THE SPASMOLYTIC ACTION OF GLUCAGON-(1–21)-PEPTIDE

As to the mechanism of action by which glucagon and glucagon-(1–21)-peptide exert their spasmolytic effects, this has not yet been fully established. It seems that in some preparations, certain arteries and veins for example, the spasmolytic action is dependent on the full sequence of glucagon. Based on present information regarding structure–activity relationships for adenylate cyclase activation, it seems that cAMP may play a central role in the spasmolytic action of glucagon in these preparations. On the other hand, in other tissues, such as the enteric smooth muscle and the biliary tree, the equipotency of glucagon and glucagon-(1–21)-peptide as far as their spasmolytic effects are concerned, indicates that they act via a mechanism which does not involve the activation of adenylate cyclase. Furthermore, the spasmolytic effect on the intestine is not potentiated by IBMX. In our hands, neither glucagon nor glucagon-(1–21)-peptide inhibited the contractions of the isolated guinea-pig ileum induced by exogenous acetylcholine, histamine, serotonin or $BaCl_2$. The observations seem to rule out the possibility of there being a direct action of glucagon or glucagon-(1–21)-peptide on the smooth muscle cells. Furthermore, alpha- and beta-adrenergic blocking agents and cholinergic blocking agents, at concentrations which, by themselves, did not influence the amplitude of contractions of the electrically stimulated guinea-pig ileum, had no influence on the spasmolytic action of glucagon nor of glucagon-(1–21)-peptide.

Prostaglandins (PGE_1 and PGE_2) are known to affect cholinergic neurotransmission[11]. At concentrations which by themselves did not induce contractions of the isolated guinea-pig ileum, prostaglandins were noted to enhance contractions induced not only by electrical stimulation but also by nicotine. Both types of contraction were effectively counteracted not only by atropine and hexamethonium but also by glucagon and glucagon-(1–21)-peptide. These findings focus on the transmission of neuronal cholinergic impulses as the site of action of glucagon and glucagon-(1–21)-peptide, and especially on the transmission through intramural cholinergic ganglia, since both nicotine and hexamethonium are considered to act mainly on ganglionic transmission. Further work is needed, however, to substantiate this suggestion of a neuronal inhibitory action of glucagon and of glucagon-(1–21)-peptide.

CONCLUSIONS

Be that as it may, the glucagon-(1–21)-peptide might emerge in the future as an alternative to glucagon in obtaining selective spasmolysis of the gastrointestinal and biliary tracts. Its clinical future will depend on whether it has less side effects than native glucagon, and/or improved pharmacokinetics, and on whether doses higher than those permitted for glucagon will show improvement of clinical efficacy.

References

1. Faloona, G. R. and Unger, R. H. (1974). Biological and immunological activity of pancreatic glucagon and enteric glucagon-like immunoreactivity. *Isr. J. Med. Sci.*, **10**, 1324
2. Lin, T. M. (1980). Gastrointestinal actions of glucagon. *Endocrinol. Jpn.*, **Sr. no. 1**, 87
3. Gagnon, G., Regoli, D. and Rioux, F. (1978). A new bioassay for glucagon. *Br. J. Pharmacol.*, **64**, 99
4. Gagnon, G., Regoli, D. and Rioux, F. (1980). Studies on the mechanism of action of glucagon in strips of rabbit renal artery. *Br. J. Pharmacol.*, **69**, 389
5. Grande, F., Grisolia, S. and Diederich, D. (1972). On the biological and chemical reactivity of carbamylated glucagon. *Proc. Soc. Exp. Biol. Med.*, **139**, 855
6. Lin,. C., Wright, D. E., Hruby, V. J. and Rodbell, M. (1975). Structure–function relationship in glucagon: properties of highly purified des-His[1]-, monoiodo-, and [des-Asn[28], Thr[29]] (homoserin lactone[27])-glucagon. *Biochemistry*, **14**, 1559
7. Rodbell, M., Birnbauer, L. and Pohl, S. L. (1971). Characteristics of glucagon action on the hepatic adenylate cyclase system. *Biochem. J.*, **125**, 58P
8. Wright, D. E., Hruby, V. J. and Rodbell, M. (1978). A reassessment of structure–function relationships in glucagon. Glucagon[1–21] is a full agonist, *J. Biol. Chem.*, **253**, 6338
9. Frandsen, E. K., Grønvald, F. C., Heding, L. G., Johansen, N. L., Lundt, B. F., Moody, A. J., Markussen, J. and Vølund, Aa. (1981). Glucagon: structure–function relationships investigated by sequence deletions. *Hoppe-Seylers Z. Physiol. Chem.*, **362**, 655
10. Assan, R. and Slusher, N. (1972). Structure/function and structure/immunoreactivity relationships of the glucagon molecule and related synthetic peptides. *Diabetes*, **21**, 843
11. Gustafsson, L., Hedqvist, P. and Lundgren, G. (1980). Pre- and post-junctional effects of prostaglandin E_2, prostaglandin synthetase inhibitors and atropine on cholinergic neurotransmission in guinea-pig ileum and bovine iris. *Acta Physiol. Scand.*, **110**, 401

Address for correspondence

Professor B. Diamant,
Novo Research Institute,
DK-2880 Bagsværd,
Denmark

DISCUSSION

Hardcastle: One of the interesting species differences with respect to glucagon is the stimulating effect it has on the dog duodenum and small bowel. I wonder if you have looked at your fragments of glucagon in respect to this. Do they have the same action?

Diamant: We have never worked with dogs in this respect. It would be interesting to find out.

Miller: I am curious to know if you have worked at all with other parts of the gastrointestinal tract, in particular, with the colon. We have found that glucagon has a different effect on stomach, duodenum, small bowel, and colon. Have you any experience with glucagon-1–21 on colon?

Diamant: Glucagon-(1–21)-peptide has the same motility inhibiting effect as glucagon on the rabbit colon, which is the only species we have studied.

Skucas: Have you looked at the esophagus of the guinea pig?

Diamant: No, not yet.

Jaspan: I am interested in the effects both of the whole glucagon molecule and of the 1–21 fragment in two situations. One you mentioned of importance, is portal vein flow as compared to renal flow, and the second is the smooth muscle effect on the renal pelvis. We observed that somatostatin can cause very marked effects on the renal pelvis, enhancing urinary flow, probably by virtue of pelviceal smooth muscle contraction. One potential clinical application of this is in renal colic with renal stones, since if it acts on the smooth muscle of the renal pelvis it might have a salutory effect in dislodging calculi. Does glucagon – either the whole molecule or the 1–21 fragment – have an effect here?

Diamant: Unfortunately I cannot say, simply because we have not yet studied the effects of these peptides on regional blood flow. It would, of course, be very interesting to do so.

Baker: I wonder about the duration of action, particularly on the bile flow, of some of the fragments that you have studied. It looked as though the time duration of the activity was about equal. Have you observed any differences with any other analogues that you may have looked at?

Diamant: No, we have not, and I will stress that we have only studied extensively the 1–21 fragment because we believed this to be the most interesting one, but I must emphasize the importance of these aspects being evaluated in man. Species differences can be very marked indeed.

Hardcastle: Have you any explanation as to why such marked species differences should exist?

Diamant: No, I really have not. It is very clear, however, that they do exist. You will recall, for example, that Lin *et al.* found glucagon-(1–21)-peptide to have no inhibitory effect on gastric acid secretion in the dog (Lin, T. M. (1980). *Endocrinol. Jpn., Sr. n° 1,* 87). We, on the other hand, have found it very effective in cats.

Hardcastle: That is true in respect to the ureter too. We found in the rabbit, for example, that it had no effect, whereas in the dog it had a profound effect.

Diamant: That is why many of the animal experiments to which people are devoting much time might prove to be of limited value; the effects seen in man may be quite different.

Miller: I can reinforce that. Dr. Chernish and some of my other colleagues and I tried somatostatin for relaxation of the stomach. In the dog this was 100 to 1000 times more effective than glucagon, whereas in man it had no effect whatsoever (Chernish, S. M. *et al.* (1981). *Am. J. Gastroenterol.*, **75**, 36).

Diamant: That is interesting. We have recently compared the effects of these two peptides on the relaxation of the guinea pig ileum and here too found somatostatin 100 times more effective than glucagon.

Jaspan: The somatostatin story is really just beginning to unfold. It now appears that an analogue, somatostatin-28, has very potent actions in insulin suppression but not in glucagon suppression. I think it would be interesting to look at this new analogue (SS-28); it seems to be very different in many ways from SS-14. There is also an SS-25, and so on. Each might well have quite different and specific actions.

Miller: I will agree with you there. On the other hand, one must not forget the very important matter of the species differences. On this point I certainly agree with Professor Diamant.

Diamant: On the subject of somatostatin, I know that in Germany it is much used in connection with gastric bleedings – in fact, it seems to be the first choice today. Do you know anything about its mode of action in this respect?

Jaspan: What it does is to drop portal vein blood flow apparently without affecting systemic, including hepatic artery, flow. In this respect it is specific for portal flow, so that it is beneficial in cases of haemorrhage from esophageal varices and peptic ulcers. The lack of systemic action is advantageous since hypotension does not occur during somatostatin infusion.

Okuda: Has anyone done a bile flow study with glucagon in cholecystectomized animals, and found an increase in the flow itself, and was there any change in the composition of bile? Because if you have the gallbladder it may relax and you do not measure the actual flow in terms of time. So, if you study the bile flow in a strict way, you have to have a cholecystectomized animal in order to measure the actual flow. Furthermore, if the bile flow increases there is a change in the composition of the bile because the portal blood may have something to do with bile flow.

Diamant: The rat, as you know, does not have a gallbladder. We have found that the bile flow in rats after the administration of glucagon and glucagon-(1–21)-peptide is enhanced compared to controls, indicating either increased production of bile or a decreased fluid absorption. Due to the absence of a gallbladder, no initial decrease occurred as noted in the guinea pig. I am sure that the experimental models could be refined very much more, but we have not done that yet.

Rey: May I come back to the metabolic effect? Working with rat liver hepatocytes and in our system of hepatocyte monolayers, we have recently tested the effect of glucagon and we have seen an increase in the influx of amino acid not metabolized, α-aminoisobutyric acid usually, and with 1–21 and 5–29 we get no action, and as you can see, it is about the same quantity that you use for spasmolytic effect and really we have no metabolic action of these analogues in our system (Figure 1).

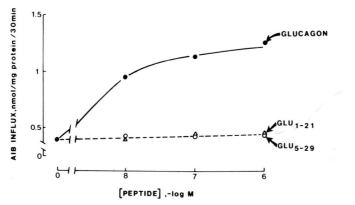

Figure 1 Effect of glucagon and of glucagon analogues GLU$_{1-21}$ and GLU$_{5-29}$ on aminoacid transport in heptocyte monolayers. (Dolais-Kitabgi, J., Lecam, A. and Rey, J.-F. (1982) INSERM U. 145 – Chemin de Vallombrose, Nice)

Diamant: That fits very nicely with our findings that these peptides do not stimulate the adenylate cyclase. The spasmolytic effect of glucagon-(1–21)-peptide must clearly be the result of some other mechanism(s).

3

The response of gastrointestinal tract motility to glucagon

R. E. MILLER and S. M. CHERNISH

INTRODUCTION

For more than thirty years prior to the isolation of glucagon, scientists had been puzzled by a temporary rise in blood sugar that sometimes followed an injection of insulin. Insulin normally reduces the amount of sugar circulating in the blood stream. Chemists, however, were unable to isolate another active compound from their insulin extracts.

Finally, in 1953, research scientists isolated and then crystallized glucagon[1,2]. It was present in such trace amounts in the pancreas of swine and cattle that 150 000 pounds of the glands were required to produce 1 ounce of active compound. Next came the even more difficult task of determining the molecular structure of glucagon. At this time the hormone had no clear-cut medical application. The primary goal of the structural studies was to gain insight into the relationship between molecular configuration and biological activity.

All proteins are composed of a number of amino acids linked in sequence. Research scientists first broke the glucagon molecule into three basic segments. Analysis of these segments revealed that the hormone contains 16 different amino acids, with a total molecular weight of 3485 daltons. Further studies showed that half of the amino acids appear more than once in the chain; simple addition showed there to be 29 in total. The realization that 8 of the hormone's 16 amino acids occur only once also proved helpful. These single units eventually served as additional reference points in a jigsaw puzzle of mammoth proportions. To give an idea of the complexity involved, there are more than 13 trillion trillion ways in which the 29 amino acids could be sequenced in a single chain. Three years of arduous effort, requiring both chemical innovations and all known methods for clarifying amino acid sequence, finally revealed the exact structure of glucagon's 473 individual atoms.

Clinical evaluation of glucagon began in 1953, shortly after its initial crystallization. The hormone quickly became a basic tool in studies of pancreatic function and of overall carbohydrate metabolism. In was first marketed in 1960 for the safe and convenient treatment of hypoglycaemic shock: the weakness or actual coma experienced by unstable diabetics when their blood sugar falls dangerously low, a problem which can be fatal if not properly treated.

Even today the hormone's complex and seemingly endless clinical possibilities continue to make it a fascinating drug for research physicians. A decade ago methods for evaluating gastrointestinal motility usually required the passage of a tube and the measurement of pressure changes within the gastrointestinal tract. Records of responses were voluminous, and difficult to interpret unless the response was 'all or nothing'. At that time our group in Indianapolis decided to try to develop radiographic techniques which were sensitive, non-invasive, and more simple to interpret. During studies of the gallbladder we noticed that glucagon relaxed not only that organ but also the duodenum. It immediately became obvious to us that glucagon may be of value in decreasing the motility and tonicity of the smooth muscle of the gastrointestinal tract.

In this paper we shall review the results of the effect of glucagon on the organs of the gastrointestinal tract as evaluated primarily during radiographic studies. Where appropriate, reference will also be made to other methods, as they pertain to the subject discussed. We shall begin with the esophagus and then proceed down the gastrointestinal tract.

ESOPHAGUS

In 1928 Wolf[3], and later Nelson[4], demonstrated varices of the esophagus radiographically. The classical features of these findings were described by Schatzki[5] and by Bediczka and Taschakert[6] in the early 1930s. The radiographic diagnosis still depends on the demonstration of (a) nodal filling defects in the distal esophagus, which may or may not be persistent, (b) widened, tortuous or worm-like mucosal folds with scalloped contours, and (c) the classic 'string of pearls' defect. Before we began our development work in this field, reports had appeared to the effect that X-ray techniques had diagnosed only some 63%, or as few as 15%, of the varices seen endoscopically[6–8]. Because of our interest in this problem we embarked upon a study to determine whether certain methods and techniques, with and without the use of drugs to enhance visualization of varices, could improve these averages[9].

Twelve volunteers, all with known varices, agreed to take part in the study. They were aged 42 to 61 years (average 52.5 years). Patients on anticoagulant therapy and those with a history of possible pheochromocytoma, insulinoma, myocardial infarction, or sensitivity or reaction to glucagon or propantheline bromide were excluded, as were those with a partial urinary bladder neck obstruction, ileus or glaucoma. None of the patients was receiving anticholinergic drugs, and no medications were given for 12 h prior to the study. The varices of the 12 patients were described as small in one patient, moderately large in three patients, very large in six, and 'enormous' in the remaining two.

The medications used in the study were placebo (2 ml of the diluting solution used for glucagon), 30 mg propantheline bromide in 2 ml of sterile water, and 2 mg glucagon similarly in 2 ml of diluent. Each medication was given intramuscularly, as a single dose, double-blind and cross-over. All patients fasted on the morning of the study. Prior to medication administration the patients were asked to empty their bladders. Prior to, and at 5, 10 and 20 minutes after the injection of the drug the patients were given two good swallows of barium. One supine (right anterior oblique to screen) and one prone (left posterior oblique to screen) after inspiration and expiration radiographs of the esophagus were obtained at each of these time periods. The patients were instructed to expectorate all saliva into a cup throughout the study in order to avoid swallowing and thus stripping the varices of blood. The patients remained lying flat on the X-ray table throughout the study.

Pulse, blood pressure and pupil size were measured before and after medication, and the patients were questioned concerning side effects. If a symptom was reported within six hours after the injection, the patient was asked to quantitate its intensity on a scale from 1 to 4 (1 for mild, 2 moderate, 3 moderately severe, and 4 severe). At the completion of the study all films were read at one sitting.

An analysis of variance was used to evaluate the responses of the patients to the three treatments. In the overall estimate of response the radiologist reported that propantheline bromide definitely helped him to visualize the esophageal varices ($p < 0.05$).

Pruszynski[8] had earlier reported that in patients with portal hypertension with varices, spasmolytic agents increased his diagnostic accuracy to 98%. Other investigators had reported excellent results when using atropine sulphate and propantheline bromide, saying that the administration of these substances enabled them to identify up to 100% of the patients who were subsequently proved to have varices[10,11].

In the presently reported study it was found: (1) that in the horizontal position maximum engorgement of the esophageal varices occurred after approximately 10 minutes, (2) that radiographs in deep expiration were superior to the inspiratory films, and (3) that the right anterior oblique view during expiration at 10 minutes was the best for diagnostic purposes. It was also noted that the esophageal varices were more easily seen after propantheline bromide than after glucagon or placebo ($p < 0.05$).

Innervation of the esophagus is primarily cholinergic[12] and contractions are inhibited by anticholinergic drugs. The esophageal peristaltic waves are unaffected by gastrointestinal hormones. This suggests that the muscles of the body of the esophagus, in contradistinction to the lower esophageal sphincter muscle, are insensitive to hormonal effects[13]. Thus, the body of the esophagus is incapable of responding to polypeptide hormones such as gastrin or glucagon. It also suggests that the enhanced visualization noted after the administration of the anticholinergic drug may be entirely secondary to the muscular relaxation of the esophageal body[14,15]. On the basis of these and of other studies in which glucagon was reported to relax the gastro-esophageal junction, Ferrucci and Long[16] evaluated the effect of glucagon in the treatment of acute food bolus impaction of the lower esophagus. Reporting on the response of six patients in whom the problem had been diagnosed by means of barium esophagoradiography, these authors found that the administration of 1 mg glucagon i.v. and the filling of the esophagus with a Column of barium enabled the food bolus to pass in most instances with complete clearing of the esophageal lumen. Marks and Lousteau[17] and Reddy[18] have reported similar findings.

Siewert et al.[19] have reported on the pressure measurements in the lower esophageal sphincter of ten patients who had clinical, radiological, and manometric evidence of achalasia. Following a single intravenous injection of 60 µg/kg body weight glucagon to these patients, and to normal subjects, these authors reported a marked and statistically significant decrease in the lower esophageal sphincter pressure lasting approximately 15 minutes. Patients with achalasia who were treated with glucagon in this way and then given a test meal ate the meal without symptoms. Previous reports of the effect of glucagon on the lower esophageal sphincter had been restricted to investigations in healthy subjects[20,21] Other than the statement that the gastro-esophageal junction is sensitive to hormonal action, the mechanism of action of glucagon on the lower esophageal sphincter remains unexplained. It is known that gastrin increases the gastro-esophageal sphincter tone[21-23] and will increase the sensitivity of the lower esophageal sphincter in patients with achalasia. This effect of gastrin on the lower esophageal sphincter can be suppressed by glucagon[21]. Siewert *et al.*[19] and Hogan *et al.*[14] have speculated that since the doses of glucagon used to induce this effect are in the pharmacological range, it is doubtful that glucagon plays a physiological role in the regulation of gastro-esophageal sphincter tone.

UPPER GASTROINTESTINAL ROENTGENOGRAPHY

In our initial study on this subject, 2 mg glucagon i.v. was compared to placebo in a double-blind and cross-over study, designed to assess the effect of glucagon on duodenal motility[24]. On that occasion it was found that the administration of glucagon resulted in a significant decrease in duodenal motility and tonicity ($p < 0.001$).

In a subsequent study 12 asymptomatic volunteers received 2 mg glucagon, 1 mg atropine sulphate, and placebo, whilst in another, 12 other volunteers received 2 mg glucagon, 30 mg propantheline bromide, and placebo intramuscularly. Both studies were double-blind and cross-over. These studies were designed to compare the effectiveness of glucagon with that of anticholinergic drugs usually used in the United States to relax the upper gastrointestinal tract[25,26].

In these studies, whilst both atropine sulphate and propantheline bromide were found to be effective ($p < 0.05$), glucagon was found to be significantly better ($p < 0.05$) than either anticholinergic for the examination of the stomach, the duodenal bulb, and the duodenal loop, and equal to them for the examination of the small bowel. One hour after the administration of the drugs, glucagon was no longer active, whereas the anticholinergic drugs still had a significant effect.

The results of these studies in control subjects have since been confirmed in patients[27,28].

Glucagon has also been used in connection with retrograde small bowel examinations. It has been reported to make the examination more comfortable for the patient; by making the small bowel more relaxed it also permits a better visualization of the lesion[29,30].

DOSE-RESPONSE STUDIES

In a dose-response study 15 volunteers, male and female, received 0.25 mg, 0.5 mg, 1 mg and 2 mg glucagon and placebo (diluting solution used for glucagon) intravenously, double-blind and cross-over[31]. In this study the effect of glucagon began after approximately 45 seconds regardless of the dose of glucagon given. There was a definite decrease ($p < 0.01$) in gastrointestinal motility and tonicity with all doses, and the dose-response was linear ($p < 0.01$).

There was atonicity of the duodenum and jejunum for an average of 8 minutes after 0.25 mg glucagon i.v., and hypotonicity lasted for an average of 12 minutes. The stomach was atonic for approximately 5 minutes and moderately hypotonic for 8.5 minutes after the same dose of glucagon. After 2 mg glucagon there was atonicity of the duodenum and jejunum for 18 minutes and moderate hypotonicity for 24 minutes; the stomach was atonic for 15 minutes and hypotonic for 22 minutes. As can be seen from these data the duration of drug effect was proportional to the size of the dose.

In a similar study 15 volunteers received the above doses of glucagon intramuscularly, double-blind and cross-over[32]. The drug effect on the duodenum and small bowel after 1 mg glucagon began after an average of 8 minutes, and lasted approximately 25 minutes. As one would expect, the onset of the effect of glucagon was slower when the drug was administered intramuscularly than when it was administered intravenously, but it tended to occur earlier as the dose of glucagon was increased.

In these studies it was found that when glucagon was given intravenously the onset of action usually occurred within 1 minute. When glucagon was given intramuscularly the onset of action ranged from 4 to 14 minutes with a more rapid onset occurring as the dose was increased. The duration of the action increased as the dose increased, regardless of the route of administration.

In a third study 15 male volunteers received placebo (diluting solution used for glucagon), 0.025 mg, 0.05 mg, 0.1 mg and 0.2 mg glucagon intravenously, double-blind and cross-over[33]. The onset of drug effect for all doses of glucagon averaged 55 seconds. The tonicity of the gastrointestinal tract was significantly decreased ($p < 0.001$) following all doses of glucagon. There was a definite linear dose response. One tenth of a milligram of glucagon induced atonicity of the stomach in 53 % of the subjects, and moderate hypotonicity in

93 % for a mean of 4.8 minutes; it induced atonicity of the duodenal loop in 93 % of the subjects, and moderate hypotonicity in 100 % for a mean of 6 minutes.

The modern short biphasic examination (air contrast plus regular examination of the stomach) is becoming more popular. A low dose of glucagon, 0.1 mg, makes this biphasic examination practical. There is no need to delay the small bowel study. Data from the above-mentioned studies indicate that the stomach is less sensitive to the action of glucagon; a dose of at least 0.1 mg intravenously or 1 mg intramuscularly is usually required before a response is seen.

HYPOTONIC COLON STUDIES

In 12 volunteers radiographic barium enema examinations of the colon were performed using 2 mg glucagon, 1 mg atropine sulphate, and placebo[34]. Medications were given intramuscularly, double-blind and cross-over. When glucagon or atrophine sulphate were given the volunteers reported less colon tonicity and increased comfort during the examination. The radiologist noted that the colon was more relaxed on the initial and the immediate post-evacuation films after glucagon and atropine sulphate than after placebo. He also reported that the intracolonic pressure was less and that the examination was more rapidly completed after glucagon than after placebo. When atropine sulphate was given *with* glucagon there was an increase in the number of reports of side effects, but the bowel relaxation was not greater than it would have been had either drug been used alone.

From previous experience[25,34] it is our impression that atropine sulphate is not as effective a relaxant of the colon as it is of the small bowel. In this study there was little measurable difference in the diameter of the normal colon before and after the active drugs were given. This is in contradistinction to what is seen in the duodenum[24,25]. These results in volunteers have since been confirmed in patients by Meeroff et al.[35], by Harned et al.[36], and by Munro[37]. As a result of these studies it is recommended that 2 mg glucagon be given intramuscularly approximately 10 minutes before beginning the barium enema examination.

Because of the excellent gastrointestinal relaxation and few reports of side effects glucagon is an excellent agent for use in hypotonic colon studies. We agree with Ferrucci and Benedict[38] that glucagon may be useful for examination of the colon in the following situations: (1) when there are lesions and diffuse painful spasm: patients with ulcerative or granulomatosis colitis or functional disorders, (2) when there are areas of localized narrowing:

patients with spasm versus constricting lesion, colonic valves or sphincters, or for the evaluation of strictures and colitis, (3) in order to decrease the smooth muscle tone of the colon for adequate distension during air contrast studies, (4) when there is a functional inability to retain enema, a situation seen more commonly in aged patients, and (5) in cases of diverticular disease, with sigmoid spasm.

RADIOGRAPHY IN INFANTS AND CHILDREN

Ratcliffe[39] has studied the use of glucagon given intravenously to infants and children during gastrointestinal radiology. He has reported that a dose of 0.5–1.0 µg/kg body weight produces satisfactory atonicity for 3–5 minutes for double contrast meals. He recommends doses of 0.8–1.25 µg/kg for barium enema examinations, and has found that such a dose given at the beginning of the examination produces atonicity for 5–10 minutes. He has stated 'The benefits of the use of these small doses of i.v. glucagon are: (1) atony, permitting good double contrast examination, (2) rapid return to normal, permitting motility to be examined, (3) relief of painful and obstructive spasm in barium enemas, (4) quietening of angry, hungry infants, (5) probable shortening of the total examination time. No undesirable side effects was observed.'

INTRALUMINAL COLON PRESSURE MEASUREMENTS

Using a three-lumen polyvinyl tube with orifices at five centimetre intervals, Chowdhury and co-workers have measured intraluminal colon pressure in the sigmoid colon, the rectum, and anal sphincter following the administration of glucagon[40,41]. In these studies glucagon was reported to have a greater inhibitory effect than secretin on food- and on morphine-induced motor activity of the distal colon and rectum. These authors concluded that in other similar studies glucagon inhibited all wave activity and significantly decreased the motility index of the hyperactive segment of the rectosigmoid junction[42]. Paul[43] and Taylor et al.[44] have measured colon myoelectrical activity and reported that glucagon inhibited both electrical and pressure rhythms in all subjects tested. The authors believe this to be due to a direct action of the drug on colonic smooth muscle.

TREATMENT OF COLON LESIONS

Other investigators have used glucagon in subjective, less well-controlled, studies for the treatment of acute diverticulitis. In one such study[45] 14 of 20 patients received 1 mg glucagon intravenously as a bolus in 10 ml of solution over a period of 8–10 minutes every 4 hours for 36 hours. The remaining six patients received 4.5 mg glucagon in 50 ml of diluent by continuous slow pump infusion over two consecutive periods of 18 hours. The authors reported that the patients had relief of symptoms within 6–24 hours (average 12 hours) after glucagon administration, together with a substantial improvement in their general condition.

In studies of ileocolic intussusception produced in 69 puppies, glucagon and hydrostatic pressure reduced 70%[46]. In this respect the difference between glucagon and placebo was not statistically significant. Cases of gangrenous intussusception were not reduced with hydrostatic pressure regardless of whether glucagon was given or not. Comparing glucagon to placebo, however, the investigators reported that when glucagon was given the reductions were significantly easier, and that there was an earlier return to normal of the vascular supply to the bowel. Fisher and Germann[47] have reported on the reduction with glucagon of intussusception in two patients who were not reduced with hydrostatic pressure alone. Hoy et al.[48] gave glucagon to 25 patients with intussusception, and reported that with glucagon and hydrostatic pressure 21 (84%) were successfully reduced.

Glucagon has also been used in conjunction with a stapling device for end-to-end anastomosis of the lower bowel[49, 50]. In these cases the spastic lower bowel is relaxed by glucagon. This allows the operator to fit the lower bowel onto the stapling device more easily and makes for a more satisfactory anastomosis. Intravenous glucagon leads to a rapid relaxation of the sigmoid colon and allows for a safer and more atraumatic anastomosis.

COMPUTED TOMOGRAPHY OF THE ABDOMEN

During CT scans of the abdomen the effect of cardiac, respiratory, and skeletal motion can be ameliorated by the computer. However, the peristaltic movement within a gas-filled viscus creates problems in the scan in that lines develop in the tomogram[51]. Because of the movement of the bowel the poorest quality scans occur in the area of the mid-abdomen. Conversely the better scans tend to be obtained in the upper abdomen and in the pelvis. Attempts to minimize the peristaltic movement have improved the scans. The drugs most often used to stop movement of the bowel are propantheline bromide and glucagon. The doses usually used for such studies have been outlined by Boldt et al.[52] Glucagon is more commonly used because it has few side effects and fewer contraindications than anticholinergic drugs. Thus, glucagon has been used for the scanning of abdominal mass lesions in children[52], abdominal pelvic tumours[53, 54], mesenteric masses[55], and for the evaluation of the pancreas[56-58]. Kirkpatrick et al.[59] have reviewed the use of glucagon in body scanning, and Kuhns et al.[60] have discussed the value of the scanning of the duodenum. CT scans of the abdomen can also be used to evaluate periaortic lymph nodes, especially in patients with Hodgkin's disease. Normal nodes can be identified in 75 % of abdominal CT scans and in 66 % of pelvic scans. This suggests that better computer programmes, machines and skill in interpretation may permit evaluation of intrinsic nodal structure in the future[61].

CHOLANGIOGRAPHY

In earlier studies glucagon was shown to relax the gallbladder[62]. In recent studies Cannon and Legge[63] have reported that glucagon relaxes the common bile duct allowing for better visualization. This is particularly important when inadequate opacification of the bile duct occurs because of an apparent obstruction or when injection of the contrast medium into the biliary system induces pain. Evans and Whitehouse[64] have reported on the use of glucagon during infusion cholangiography. They have noted that there is an increased likelihood of obtaining good visualization of the gallbladder after the administration of glucagon. Thus, when the gallbladder is not opacified on glucagon augmented cholangiography, it reinforces the diagnosis of probably significant gallbladder disease.

The distal portion of the common bile duct can be difficult to visualize especially if it is not dilated, despite the increase in resolution of modern grey scale ultrasonic equipment[65]. In a recent series only 38 % of cases with non-obstructive jaundice demonstrated the common bile duct[66]. The posterior relationship of the common bile duct to the generally gas-filled duodenal bulb results in its poor ultrasonic visualization. The upper intestinal gas can be at least partially eliminated with the use of oral water. However, the water continues to leave the stomach as the stomach contracts constantly. When glucagon is given peristalsis ceases within approximately 30 to 45 seconds and remains absent for 6 to 15 minutes. Pon and Cooperberg have reported that the use of water and glucagon has improved their ability to demonstrate the distal common bile duct[65].

EXPULSION OF IMPACTED CALCULI INTO THE DUODENUM

Impacted calculi in the distal common duct are difficult to engage with a basket and can be responsible for the failure of the steerable catheter technique. Many techniques have been described for proximal relocation of impacted calculi, but all have had little success. The list includes the use of the Trendelenburg position, suction, flushing, irrigation, Foley catheters, forceps, choledochoscopes, basket manoeuvres, and chemical dissolution. Because of ampullary spasm, small and even some large (6 mm) stones can be pushed through the ampulla vater into the duodenum after an intravenous injection of glucagon[67]. The relaxation of the distal choledochal sphincter has permitted the non-operative removal of retained common duct calculi. This method has proved successful when percutaneous stone removal has failed. The amount of glucagon used was 1 mg intravenously.

ENDOSCOPY

Glucagon is not indicated during the usual endoscopic procedures for study of the upper gastrointestinal tract except in the following circumstances: (1) when there is marked or excessive motility of the gastric antrum and pylorus and one wishes to obtain good photographs of that area[68–71], (2) when one wishes to decrease or stop gastric movement in order to remove a polyp[70,72], (3) when one is unable to adequately view the duodenum[69,72–74], (4) when one is trying to obtain a biopsy of an ulcer and there is excessive movement of the gastric antrum[68,71,72], (5) when one is trying to remove a foreign body from the stomach[72], and (6) during retrograde pancreatography or cholangiography, when glucagon given intravenously will stop duodenal movement and allow the passage of the catheter into the sphincter of Oddi for better visualization of the pancreatic and/or biliary ducts[72,73,75,76]. During colonoscopy glucagon may be given when removal of polyps is contemplated. This allows the colon to relax when the polyp is being encircled. By relaxing the colon, glucagon also helps to prevent the walls of the colon coming together when the current is applied to cut off the polyp, a situation which can result in perforation of the colon.

IN SUMMARY

Glucagon is a molecule with 29 amino acids and a molecular weight of 3485 daltons. It was originally isolated and crystallized in 1953 and was first made available in 1960 for the treatment of hypoglycaemia in diabetic patients.

In 1972 it was reported to relax the gallbladder, stomach, duodenum, duodenal bulb and small bowel during radiography; in 1974 it was reported to relax the colon, and in 1976 the gastroesophageal junction. These findings opened the way for further studies by many investigators.

It has been found useful in a dose of 0.1 mg, given intravenously, to relax the stomach, duodenal bulb, duodenum and small bowel during the modern short biphasic examination (air contrast plus regular examination of the stomach). This low dose makes the biphasic examination practical because the short duration of action of this dose of glucagon allows the study of the small bowel to proceed without delay.

Glucagon has also proved useful in the upper gastrointestinal tract during endoscopy by facilitating the procedure. During CT examinations of the abdomen relaxation of the upper gastrointestinal tract has eliminated disturbing lines in the scans improving the quality of the scans of the liver, spleen and pancreas. In ultrasonography of the gallbladder the common bile duct can be better visualized if seen through a background of water. Glucagon eliminates duodenal peristalsis and allows the gas-filled duodenum to be filled with water for better common bile duct visualization.

Glucagon also relaxes the colon, allowing the radiologist to complete a more comfortable examination for the patient. It decreases painful spasm and facilitates decision-making concerning areas of localized narrowing, spasm versus constricting lesions, colonic valves and sphincters, and the evaluation of strictures and colitis. Glucagon decreases smooth muscle tone helping the patient to retain the enema and allows for adequate distension during air contrast studies.

During colonoscopy glucagon has been found to be of value by relaxing the colon prior to polypectomy; it is easier to apply a snare to a polyp in a stilled colon, and its use also reduces the risk of perforation caused by the walls of the colon coming together when the current is applied.

References

1. Staub, A., Sinn, L. and Behrens, O. K. (1953). Purification and crystallization of hyperglycemic glucogenolytic factor (HGF). *Science*, **117**, 628
2. Staub, A., Sinn, L. and Behrens, O. K. (1955). Purification and crystallization of glucagon. *J. Biol. Chem.*, **214**, 619
3. Wolf, G. (1928). Erkennung von Oesophagus. Varizen mit Röntgenbilder. *Fortschr. Röntgenstr.*, **37**, 890
4. Nelson, S. W. (1957). Roentgenographic diagnosis of esophageal varices. *Am. J. Roentgenol.*, **77**, 599
5. Schatzki, R. (1931). Die Röntgendiagnose der Oesophagus- und Magenvarizen und ihre Bedeutung für die Klinik. *Fortschr. Rötgenstr.*, **44**, 28
6. Bediczka, I. G. and Taschakert, J. (1932). Die Röntgenologische Diagnostik der Oesophagusvarizen. *Fortschr. Röntgenstr.*, **46**, 156
7. Atkins, J. P. (1963). Varices of esophagus. In Bochus, H. L. (ed.) *Gastroenterology*, second edition, p. 224 (Philadelphia: W. B. Saunders)
8. Pruszynski, B. (1969). Zastosowanie silnie dzialajacych środków rozkurczowych w retngenodiagnostyce żylaków przelyku. *Pol. Przegl. Radiol.*, **33**, 73

9. Cockerill, E. M., Miller, R. E., Chernish, S. M., McLaughlin, G. C. and Rodda, B. E. (1976). Optimal visualization of esophageal varices. *Am. J. Roentgenol.*, **126**, 512

10. Dalinka, M. K., Smith, E. H., Wolfe, R. D., Goldenberg, D. and Langdon, D. E. (1972). Pharmacologically enhanced visualization of esophageal varices by Pro-Banthine. Preliminary report. *Radiology*, **102**, 281

11. Ghahremani, G. C., Port, R. B., Winans, C. S. and Williams, J. R. Jr. (1972). Esophageal varices. Enhanced radiological visualization by anticholinergic drugs. *Am. J. Dig. Dis.*, **17**, 703

12. Adam, C. W. M., Brain, R. F. H., Ellis, F. G., Kaintze, R. and Trounce, J. R. (1961). Achalasia of cardia. *Guy's Hosp. Rep.*, **110**, 191

13. Cohn, S. (1975). Symptomatic diffuse esophageal spasm and its relation to gastrin hypersensitivity. (Editorial) *Ann. Intern. Med.*, **82**, 714

14. Hogan, W. J., Dodds, W. J., Hoke, S. E., Reid, D. P., Kalkhoff, R. K. and Arndorfer, R. C. (1975). Effect of glucagon on esophageal motor function. *Gastroenterology*, **69**, 160

15. Hollis, J. B., Levine, S. M. and Castell, D. O. (1972). Differential sensitivity of human esophagus to pentagastrin. *Am. J. Physiol.*, **122**, 870

16. Ferrucci, J. T. and Long, J. A., Jr. (1977). Radiologic treatment of esophageal food impaction using intravenous glucagon. *Radiology*, **125**, 25

17. Marks, H. W. and Lousteau, R. J. (1979). Glucagon and esophageal meat impaction. *Arch. Otolaryngol.*, **105**, 367

18. Reddy, A. N. (1981). Noninvasive management of esophageal meat impaction. *Gastrointest. Endosc.*, **27**, 202

19. Siewert, R., Früh, E. and Waldeck, F. (1973). Pressure decrease in the lower esophageal sphincter in achalasia by glucagon. *Germ. Med. Mon.*, **3**, 107

20. Jaffer, S. S., Makhlouf, G. M., Alonso, B. A. and Zfass, A. M. (1973). Kinetics of inhibition of lower esophageal sphincter pressure by glucagon. *Gastroenterology*, **64**, 860

21. Waldeck, F., Siewert, R., Jennewein, H. M. and Weiser, F. (1973). Das Druckprofil im unteren Ösophagussphinkter beim Menschen und seine Beeinflussung durch Gastrin, Calcitonin und Glucagon. *Dtsch. Med. Wschr.*, **98**, 1059

22. Cohen, S. and Lipschutz, W. (1971). Hormonal regulation of human lower esophageal sphincter competence. Interaction of gastrin and secretin. *J. Clin. Invest.*, **50**, 449

23. Jennewein, H. M., Waldeck, F. and Prahl, K. (1972). Zur Beeinflussung des unteren Oseophagussphinkters durch gastrointestinale Hormone biem Hund. *Leber-Magen-Darm*, **2**, 17

24. Chernish, S. M., Miller, R. E., Rosenak, B. D. and Scholz, N. E. (1972). Hypotonic duodenography with use of glucagon. *Gastroenterology*, **63**, 392

25. Miller, R. E., Chernish, S. M., Rosenak, B. D. and Rodda, B. E. (1973). Hypotonic duodenography with glucagon. *Radiology*, **108**, 35

26. Miller, R. E., Chernish, S. M., Skucas, J., Rosenak, B. D. and Rodda, B. E. (1974). Hypotonic roentgenology with glucagon. *Am. J. Roentgenol.*, **121**, 264

27. Bertrand, G., Linscheer, W. G., Raheja, K. L. and Woods, R. E. (1977). Double-blind evaluation of glucagon and propantheline bromide (Pro-Banthine) for hypotonic duodenography. *Am. J. Roentgenol.*, **128**, 197

28. Carsen, G. M. and Finby, N. (1976). Hypotonic duodenography with glucagon. Clinical comparison study. *Radiology*, **118**, 529

29. Miller, R. E. and Lehman, G. (1972). Localization of small bowel hemorrhage. Complete reflux small bowel examination. *Am. J. Dig. Dis.*, **17**, 1019

30. Hecht, H. L., Hollenberg, G. M. and Pradhan, A. R. (1979). Glucagon-induced small intestine hypotonia demonstrating bleeding lymphoma. *Gastrointest. Radiol.*, **4**, 61

31. Miller, R. E., Chernish, S. M., Brunelle, R. L. and Rosenak, B. D. (1978). Double-blind radiographic study of dose response to intravenous glucagon for hypotonic duodenography. *Radiology*, **127**, 55

32. Miller, R. E., Chernish, S. M., Brunelle, R. L. and Rosenak, B. D. (1978). Dose response to

intramuscular glucagon during hypotonic radiography. *Radiology*, **127**, 49

33. Miller, R. E., Chernish, S. M., Greenman, G. F., Maglinte, D. D. T., Rosenak, B. D. and Brunelle, R. L. (1982). Radiography with small dose glucagon. *Radiology* (In press)

34. Miller, R. E., Chernish, S. M., Skucas, J., Rosenak, B. D. and Rodda, B. E. (1974). Hypotonic colon examination with glucagon. *Radiology*, **113**, 555

35. Meeroff, J. C., Jorgens, J. and Isenberg, J. I. (1975). The effect of glucagon on barium enema examination. *Radiology*, **115**, 5

36. Harned, R. K., Stelling, C. B., Williams, S. and Wolf, G. L. (1976). Glucagon and barium enema examinations. A controlled clinical trial. *Am. J. Roentgenol.*, **126**, 981

37. Munro, T. G. (1979). Pit falls to avoid. Spasm in ulcerative colitis masquerading as carcinoma. *J. Can. Assoc. Radiol.*, **30**, 171

38. Ferrucci, J. T., Jr. and Benedict, K. T., Jr. (1971). Anti-cholinergic-aided study of gastrointestinal tract. *Radiol. Clin. N. Am.*, **9**, 23

39. Ratcliffe, J. F. (1980). Glucagon in barium examinations in infants and children. Special reference to dosage. *Br. J. Radiol.*, **53**, 860

40. Chowdhury, A. R. and Lorber, S. H. (1974). Effects of glucagon and secretin on food or morphine-induced motor activity of the distal colon, rectum, and anal sphincter. *Am. Fed. Clin. Res.*, **22**, 693

41. Chowdhury, A. R., Dinoso, V. and Lorber, S. H. (1976). Characterization of hyperactive segment of the rectosigmoid junction. *Gastroenterology*, **71**, 584

42. Chowdhury, A. R. and Lorber, S. H. (1977). Effects of glucagon and secretin on food or morphine induced motor activity of the distal colon, rectum, and anal sphincter. *Am. J. Dig. Dis.*, **22**, 775

43. Paul, F. (1974). Quantitative Untersuchungen der Wirking von Pankreasglukagon und Sekretin auf die Magen-Darm-Motorik mittels elektromanometrischer Simultanregistrierungen beim Menschem. *Klin. Wschr.*, **52**, 983

44. Taylor, I., Duthie, H. L., Cumberland, D. C. and Smallwood, R. (1975). Glucagon and the colon. *Gut*, **16**, 973

45. Daniel, O., Basu, P. K. and Al-Samarrae, H. M. (1974). Use of glucagon in the treatment of acute diverticulitis. *Br. Med. J.*, **3**, 720

46. Haase, G. M. and Boles, E. T., Jr. (1979). Glucagon in experimental intussusception. *J. Ped. Surg.*, **14**, 664

47. Fisher, J. K. and Germann, D. R. (1977). Glucagon-aided reduction of intussusception. *Radiology*, **122**, 197

48. Hoy, G. R., Dunbar, D. and Boles, E. T., Jr. (1977). The use of glucagon in the diagnosis and management of ileocolic intussusception. *J. Ped. Surg.*, **12**, 939

49. Harford, F. J., Jr. (1979). Use of glucagon in conjunction with the end-to-end anastomosis (EEA) stapling device for low anterior anastomoses. *Dis. Colon. Rect.*, **22**, 452

50. Moseson, M. D., Hoexter, B. and Labow, S. D. (1980). Glucagon, a useful adjunct in anastomosis with a stapling device. *Dis. Colon Rect.*, **23**, 25

51. Alfidi, R. J., MacIntyre, W. J. and Haaga, J. R. (1976). The effects of biological motion on CT resolution. *Am. J. Roentgenol.*, **127**, 11

52. Boldt, D. W. and Reilly, D. J. (1977). Computed tomography of abdominal mass lesions in children. *Radiology*, **124**, 371

53. von Fotter, R. and Sager, W. D. (1979). CT des Beckens und Abdomens im Kindesalter. *Fortschr. Röntgenstr.*, **131**, 476

54. von Fotter, R., Sager, W. D., Justich, E. and Nedden, D. (1980). Zur Bedeutung der Computertomographie in der pädiatrischen Diagnostik abdomineller und pelviner tumoren. *Röntgen-Bl.*, **33**, 156

55. Bernardino, M. E., Jing, B. S. and Wallace, S. (1979). Computed tomography diagnosis of mesenteric masses. *Am. Roentgen. Ray Soc.*, **132**, 33

56. Stanley, R. J., Sagel, S. S. and Lefitt, R. G. (1977). Computed tomographic evaluation of the

pancreas. *Radiology*, **124**, 715

57. Modder, U., Friedmann, G., Büchelar, E., Baert, F., Lackner, C., Brecht, G., Buurmann, R., Rupp, N. and Heller, H. J. (1979). Werte und Ergebnisse der Computertomographie bei Pankreaserkrankungen. *Fortschr. Röntgenstr.*, **130**, 57

58. Moss, A. A., Kressel, H. Y., Korobkin, M., Goldberg, H. I., Rohlfing, D. M. and Brasch, R. C. (1978). The effect of gastrografin and glucagon on CT scanning of the pancreas. A blind clinical trial. *Radiology*, **126**, 711

59. Kirkpatrick, R. H., Wittenberg, J., Schaffer, D. L., Black, E. B., Hall, D. A., Braitman, B. S. and Ferrucci, J. T., Jr. (1978). Scanning techniques in computed body tomography. *Am. J. Roentgenol.*, **130**, 1069

60. Kuhns, L. R., Seigel, R., Borlaza, G. and Rapp, R. (1979). Visualization of the longitudinal fold of the duodenum by computed tomography. *J. Comp. Assist. Tomogr.*, **3**, 345

61. Redman, H. C., Federal, W. A., Castellino, R. A. and Glatstein, E. (1977). Evaluation of normal and abnormal lymph nodes at computerized tomographic scanning of the abdomen and pelvis. Presented at the *First European Seminar on Computerized Axial Tomography in Clinical Practice.*

62. Chernish, S. M., Miller, R. E., Rosenak, B. D. and Scholz, N. E. (1972). Effect of glucagon on size of visualized human gallbladder before and after a fat meal. *Gastroenterology*, **62**, 1218

63. Cannon, P. and Legge, D. (1979). Glucagon as a hypotonic agent in cholangiography. *Clin. Radiol.*, **30**, 49

64. Evans, A. F. and Whitehouse, G. H. (1979). The effect of glucagon on infusion cholangiography. *Clin. Radiol.*, **30**, 499

65. Pon, M. S. and Cooperberg, P. L. (1979). Oral water and intravenous glucagon to aid ultrasonic visualization of the common bile duct. *J. Can. Assoc. Radiol.*, **30**, 174

66. Sample, W. F., Sarti, D. A. and Goldstein, L. I. (1978). Gray-scale ultrasonography of the jaundiced patient. *Radiology*, **128**, 719

67. Latshaw, R. F., Kadir, S., Witt, W. S., Kaufman, S. L. and White, R. I. (1981). Glucagon induced choledochal sphincter relaxation. Aid for expulsion of impacted calculi into the duodenum. *Am. J. Radiol.*, **137**, 614

68. Hradsky, M., Stockbrügger, R. and Ostberg, H. (1973). The effect of glucagon on gastric motility, the pylorus, and reflux of bile into the stomach during gastroscopic examination. *Scand. J. Gastroenterol.*, **8** (suppl. 20), 26 (Abstract)

69. Bertrand, G., Woods, R. E., Raheja, K. L. and Linscheer, W. G. (1975). Double blind evaluation of two hypotonic drugs for duodenoscopy and duodenography. *Gastroenterology*, **68**, 1069 (Abstract)

70. Hradsky, M. and Furugard, K. (1976). Electrosurgical gastric polypectomy and duodenoscopy with the use of glucagon – Novo. *Scand. J. Gastroenterol.*, **11**, 54 (Abstract)

71. Kiil, J., Andersen, D. and Weinreich, J. (1976). A double-blind comparison of gastric relaxation after buscopan and glucagon – Novo. *Scand. J. Gastroenterol.*, **11** (suppl. 38), 58 (Abstract)

72. Paul, F., Misaki, F. and Seifert, E. (1973). Crystalline pancreatic glucagon. A new spasmolytic agent. Results of comparative endoscopic and electromanometric investigations in the proximal gastro-intestinal tract. *Endoscopy*, **5**, 199

73. Hradsky, M., Furugard, K., Stockbrügger, R. and Dotevall, G. (1974). The use of glucagon during upper gastrointestinal endoscopy. *Scand. J. Gastroenterol.*, **9** (suppl. 27), 48 (Abstract)

74. Mlecko, L. M. (1974). Hypotonic duodenoscopy using glucagon. *Gastroenterology*, **66**, 818 (Abstract)

75. Silvis, S. E. and Vennes, J. A. (1975). The role of glucagon in endoscopic cholangiopancreatography. *Gastrointest. Endosc.*, **21**, 162

76. Nebel, O. T. (1973). Therapeutic endoscopic pancreatocholangiogram. *U.S. Navy Med.*, **61**, 25

Address for correspondence

Professor R. E. Miller, Indiana University Medical Center, Department of Radiology, 1100 West Michigan Street, Indianapolis, IN 46223, USA

DISCUSSION

Hardcastle: With the very low levels of glucagon you have given, 0.025 mg, have you any idea what blood levels you obtain, as these blood levels might suggest that glucagon could have a physiological role in the gastrointestinal tract.

Miller: We have not checked blood levels following the administration of these very low doses of glucagon; I can simply report that the patients suffered no side effects. In an earlier study (not yet published) we did check blood levels in healthy volunteers given doses of 1 or 2 mg glucagon. The volunteers themselves could detect no differences between the two doses; the blood levels after both doses were higher than normal.

Hardcastle: But you spoke of one patient who was worried about the examination because he had dilated duodenum. Would that not suggest to you that the glucagon might have had a physiological role?

Miller: Glucagon is, of course, a 'stress hormone', and if the patient is at all anxious or nervous his own glucagon level will rise even before you administer exogenous glucagon to him. For this reason in some instances the glucagon level will rise following an injection of placebo. This fact sometimes leads people erroneously to conclude that no glucagon is needed. In the colon examination, if you stress the patient enough, you can make a good examination. The patient will be exceedingly uncomfortable and he will use his own glucagon, but, of course, this is not necessarily the proper way to do the examination.

Jaspan: In my experience the normal response to stress is that the glucagon level will increase from about 100 pg/ml to a maximum of 400–600 pg/ml. This, I would suggest, is a pharmacologic action. If you inject 1 mg as a bolus you get about 10 000 pg/ml (10 ng) which decreases rapidly. A 0.1 mg bolus dose will give you a peak blood level of around 1500 to 2000 pg/ml, which is about ten times the physiologic level. I would think that while you might get at maximum stress a borderline effect, the effects that we are seeing are in the pharmacologic or high physiologic range of glucagon. The 1 and 2 mg doses used earlier were horrendously high. I think that a clear-cut differentiation must be made between the physiologic actions, which are receptor mediated and adenyl cyclase dependent, and most of the actions about which we have talked today, which I think are not receptor mediated nor adenyl cyclase dependent, but rather a direct action of supraphysiologic levels of the hormone on whatever target organ they are acting.

Hardcastle: But it would appear that you can get actions on the gastrointestinal tract which are at the top limit of the physiological range.

Jaspan: In certain instances, such as portal blood flow, this may well be the case. However, many other factors are probably superimposed on the meal stimulated increase in portal blood flow. The effects on portal blood flow after a bolus injection are, I would guess, much greater than those due to physiologic hyperglucagonaemia after a meal.

Christiansen: How long does it take, when you are using a barium enema, to advance the contrast into the small intestine?

Miller: It is much more rapid than the usual small bowel examination. The usual examination, giving barium by mouth, can take anywhere from 20 minutes to 5 hours. By instilling barium through the rectum until it reaches the ileocecal valve or terminal ileum, or even the duodenum, the examination can be completed very speedily, in say 4–5 minutes, or 15 minutes at the most. The saving in time is obviously advantageous, particularly if the patient is in a poor condition and is found to need operating upon right away in order to avoid large blood loss or things of that nature. This is clearly a good way of rapidly coming to a firm diagnosis.

Okuda: Can you tell us a little more about the potential use of glucagon in the management of impacted gallstones? How many cases have you studied, and what is the largest size you have expelled?

Miller: To my knowledge there have been three reported cases of 6 mm stones being pushed into the duodenum. Burhenne was the first to use this technique; using baskets, he succeeded in pushing 3 mm stones through the choledochus (Burhenne, H. J. (1973). *AJR*, **117**, 388). Recently it has been reported that 6 mm stones have been pushed through the choledochus, or the sphincter of Oddi, after glucagon when it was not possible before (Latshaw, R. F. *et al.* (1981). *AJR*, **137**, 614). I can see that this idea may cause concern to some people, in that they might be worried that the stones would be pushed through the duct and cause a fistula. I think that the risk of this happening depends on the skill of the operator. He must appreciate that when using glucagon he cannot use extra force. With glucagon the choledochus relaxes and the stones can be pushed through.

Rey: To be honest, I am not really sure that some of the reports about stones being passed through the papilla, even with glucagon, are very accurate. It seems to me quite likely, unless of course one has endoscopic control, that one sometimes passes through spontaneous or provoked fistulae between the infundibulum and the duodenum. This is something known to everyone doing ERCP and endoscopic sphincterotomy.

Miller: That may well be. What I am doing today is reporting to you some recent cases where stones larger than 3 mm were pushed through after giving glucagon. Some radiologists say (Burhenne, personal communication) that you should stop at 3 mm stones, others report that they have pushed 6 mm stones through quite successfully. I do not know the answer. All I do know is that glucagon relaxes the papilla, thus facilitating the manoeuvre.

4

On the use of glucagon—ancillary effects and other considerations

R. E. MILLER and S. M. CHERNISH

When chemists began work on determining the nature of the hypoglycaemic material associated with insulin, it is doubtful that they envisioned that the substance they were investigating, subsequently called glucagon, would one day prove to have a use in so many areas of medicine. Even when work was begun on its synthesis, it is unlikely that much thought was given to the possible use of this substance in clinical medicine. The aim of the present book is to elucidate the usefulness of glucagon; in this chapter we plan to explore the side effects, ancillary effects, and other considerations of its use as a diagnostic agent of gastrointestinal lesions.

SIDE EFFECTS

The side effects of glucagon have been reviewed[1] on the basis of seven studies in which the drug was given intramuscularly and two in which it was given intravenously. All nine studies were conducted by the same team, and the doses used were the same throughout. In all instances, bar one, the studies were carried out in healthy volunteers; the one exception was a study conducted in patients with esophageal varices. The studies were of a double-blind, cross-over design, and barium was given either orally or by enema.

Taking first the studies in which the medications were administered intramuscularly, a total of 87 subjects received placebo and 2 mg glucagon, 48 received 1 mg atropine sulphate, and 36 received 30 mg propantheline bromide. Subjects indicating the occurrence of a complaint after the administration of the various substances were asked to rate its intensity on a scale from 1 to 4: 1 for mild, 2 for moderate, 3 for moderately severe, and 4 for severe. The complaints reported are shown in Table 1. (Those mentioned only once are grouped together under 'miscellaneous'.) Because of the unequal numbers of subjects receiving each of the medications, the data in Table 1 are recorded under the headings 'percent frequency' and 'average intensity'. The 'percent frequency' figures are the percentage calculations of the number of reports of each complaint divided by the number of subjects receiving each medication. The 'average intensity' figures are the results of dividing the total score for intensity by the number of subjects experiencing each complaint. In each study a fair number of subjects reported the occurrence of more than one complaint; this was particularly so in the case of the anticholinergic drugs.

After the intramuscular administration of glucagon the percent frequency of all complaints was 54% with an average intensity of 1.8, after propantheline bromide it was 86.1% with an average intensity of 2.3, after atropine sulphate 93.8% with an average intensity of 1.9, and after placebo 33.3% with an average intensity of 1.3. Thus, approximately one-third of those given placebo and one-half of those given glucagon reported a side effect that was mild to moderate, whereas higher percentages of subjects given anticholinergic drugs reported side effects with an average intensity of moderate to moderately severe. A review of the data given in Table 1 shows a tendency for glucagon to be associated with nausea and vomiting, atropine sulphate with dryness of the mouth, and propantheline bromide with nausea, abdominal distress, dry mouth, headache, blurring of vision and urinary difficulties. The 33.3% incidence of side effects following the administration of placebo suggests that there is some unavoidable discomfort when undergoing the average radiological diagnostic procedure.

The complaints occurring after the intravenous administration of placebo and glucagon are shown in Table 2. When placebo was given the percent frequency of reports for all complaints was 11.1% and the average intensity was mild. When glucagon was given the percent frequency was 51.9% with an average intensity of mild to moderate. Again, nausea was reported more often after glucagon than after placebo.

Pulse and blood pressure rates were measured with the subjects sitting, prior to and approximately one hour after the administration of medication. When the figures following the administration of glucagon, both intramuscular and

Table 1 Percentage of reports and average intensity[a] of complaints reported by volunteers given each medication intramuscularly

Complaint	Placebo (87)[b]		Atropine sulphate (48)		Propantheline bromide (36)		Glucagon (87)	
	% freq.	Average intensity	% freq.	Average intensity	% freq.	Average intensity	% freq.	Average intensity
Nausea	6.9	1.5	14.6	1.3	36.1[c]	1.5	36.8[c]	2.0
Vomiting	1.1	1.0	2.1	1.0	8.3	1.7	13.8[d]	1.4
Abdominal distress	9.2	1.5	20.8	1.2	36.1[d]	1.7	10.3	1.8
Diarrhoea	1.1	1.0	0	—	0	—	4.6	2.3
Dry mouth	13.8	1.2	89.6[c]	2.3	83.3[c]	3.2	13.8	1.5
Sore throat	0	—	2.1	2.0	2.8	4.0	0	—
Headache	6.9	1.0	16.7	1.6	30.6[d]	1.5	6.9	2.0
Dizziness	6.9	1.3	4.2	1.0	13.9	1.6	8.0	1.9
Lightheadedness	1.1	3.0	0	—	0	—	3.4	1.3
Drowsiness	0	—	4.2	2.0	5.6	1.5	1.1	4.0
Feeling flushed	0	—	2.1	2.0	16.7[e]	1.8	3.4	1.7
Perspiration	2.3	1.0	4.2	2.0	0	—	4.6	1.0
Blurred vision	0	—	0	—	13.9	2.8	0	—
Dysuria	1.1	2.0	2.1	1.0	13.9	2.6	1.1	1.0
Bladder discomfort	0	—	0	—	8.3	1.7	0	—
Difficult urination	0	—	0	—	16.7	1.8	0	—
Urinary retention	0	—	0	—	27.8[d]	3.7	0	—
Miscellaneous	1.2	2.0	6.3	2.3	25.0	2.3	1.2	1.0
% Frequency of all reports	33.3		93.8[c]		86.1[e]		54.0[d]	
Average intensity		1.3		1.9		2.3		1.8

[a] 0–none, 1–mild, 2–moderate, 3–moderately severe, and 4–severe
[b] Numbers in parentheses indicate number of subjects given the drug
[c] $p < 0.001$ when drug is compared to placebo
[d] $p < 0.01$
[e] $p < 0.05$

(Miller, R. E. et al., 1979. Reprinted, with permission, from Gastrointest. Radiol., **4**, 1)

Table 2 Percentage of reports and average intensity[a] of complaints reported by volunteers given each medication intravenously

Complaint	Placebo (27)[b]		Glucagon 2 mg (27)	
	% freq.	Average intensity	% freq.	Average intensity
Nausea	7.4	1.0	44.4	1.8
Abdominal distress	3.7	1.0	3.7	1.0
Diarrhoea			3.7	1.0
Dry mouth	3.7	1.0		
Headache			14.8	1.8
Dizziness			7.4	1.5
Feeling flushed			3.7	1.0
Tinnitus			3.7	1.0
% frequency of all reports	11.1		51.9	
Average intensity		1.0		1.6

[a] 1 – mild, 2 – moderate, 3 – moderately severe, and 4 – severe
[b] Numbers in parentheses indicate numbers of subjects given the drug

(Miller, R. E. *et al.*, 1979. Reprinted, with permission, from *Gastrointest. Radiol.*, **4**, 1)

intravenous, were compared to placebo, no changes were seen which could be attributed to the medication. When compared to placebo or to glucagon, the administration of atropine sulphate, however, was found to be associated with an increase in the pulse rate of approximately 16 beats per minute ($p < 0.05$); propantheline bromide was found to be associated with an increase of approximately 35 beats per minute, an increase which was significantly greater ($p < 0.05$) than that seen following the administration of atropine sulphate. Similarly, the diastolic blood pressure rates after the administration of the anticholinergic drugs were significantly higher ($p < 0.05$) than after the administration of placebo or of glucagon.

The results of these studies suggest that in this volunteer population and small group of patients undergoing diagnostic radiographic procedures, reports of side effects were few and mild when glucagon or placebo were given. When, however, the subjects received anticholinergic drugs there was a definite increase in reports of moderate to moderately severe side effects, and the pulse rate and diastolic blood pressure rates also increased.

In a letter recently published in the *Journal of the American Medical Association*, Levenstein[2] reported the case of a 78-year-old woman who received 0.5 mg glucagon intravenously for a double contrast upper gastrointestinal examination. Thirty minutes later the patient reported dizziness and abdominal cramping and abruptly lost consciousness. When she awoke 2 minutes later her right arm was paretic and there was right central facial paresis. Her blood pressure at that stage was recorded as 100/60 mmHg. During the next $\frac{1}{2}$ hour she had 10 liquid stools. Ninety minutes after the contrast study her BP was 160/80, there was no abdominal pain, and the hemiparesis had completely resolved. Levenstein believes that the patient experienced a syndrome of low-flow through arteriosclerotic cerebral vessels as a consequence of glucagon-induced intestinal fluid pooling and diarrhoea.

The diarrhoea is difficult to explain, although this complaint was reported by three subjects in one of the double-blind cross-over studies mentioned earlier[3]. (One subject reported one watery stool after 0.25 mg glucagon as mild, one reported one watery stool after 1 mg glucagon as moderately severe, and one reported four watery stools after 2 mg glucagon as mild.) As these subjects had each received different doses of the drug there was no evidence of a dose-related response. Overall, diarrhoea was an uncommon complaint in the studies mentioned earlier; its frequency was 5% and its intensity moderate[1].

When Barbezat and Grossman[4–6] studied the effect of glucagon and gastrin on gastrointestinal fluid in dogs, they reported that the administration of these two substances resulted in a stimulation of fluid from the jejunum and ileum of dogs with Thiry-Vella loops. Neither hormone alone caused diarrhoea, but when the two hormones were given together there was profuse watery diarrhoea in all five of the authors' tests. No good explanation was offered as to why this should have occurred. In all of these tests the hormones were given continuously by intravenous infusion, whereas a bolus dose is given for gastrointestinal radiology.

Hicks and Turnberg[7], working with humans, reported that in their studies an intravenous infusion of glucagon reduced jejunal absorption of sodium, chloride and water. They reported a watery diarrhoea after doses of 0.3 µg/kg per hour of glucagon, and perfusion of the intestine with saline. Interestingly as the dose of glucagon was increased its effect on ion transport decreased. Apparently the difference in response between the two studies is caused by the perfusion of the intestine by Hicks and Turnberg[7] with a saline solution. Mallinson et al.[8] reported on 9 patients with glucagonoma syndrome. Intermittent diarrhoea with hypokalaemia occurred in 6 of these 9 patients with relapse of the rash. These patients had elevated levels of plasma glucagon and had imbided food and fluids. Patients reporting to the radiology department for gastrointestinal studies, however, have normally fasted for 12 hours and not taken fluids since the previous midnight.

Without additional information it is difficult to judge the cause of the diarrhoea in the case reported by Levenstein[2]. However, on the basis of the studies discussed above one wonders if the patient may have had increased levels of plasma gastrin. The addition of glucagon to a patient with increased levels of gastrin could indeed result in abdominal distress and marked watery diarrhoea. In addition some radiologists administer cold saline after an upper gastrointestinal study in order to speed the small intestinal transit; this could also be a cause of diarrhoea[9, 10].

A small quantity of lactose, approximately 24.5 mg, is given with every 0.5 mg of glucagon. Lactose, given orally and in much larger quantities, does indeed sometimes cause diarrhoea and abdominal distress in susceptible patients. We do not believe, however, that small quantities given intravenously would be likely to cause a similar problem, even in susceptible patients.

The course of events of this patient's symptoms other than the diarrhoea and abdominal distress suggests vasodepressor syncope[11]. The most familiar example of syncope is the common faint. It stems from a sudden and precipitous fall in peripheral resistance, probably involving both arterioles and veins, accompanied by an increase in cardiac output that usually follows peripheral vasodilatation. The patient becomes pale, breaks out in a cold sweat, and complains of nausea. At this time he may also experience chills and shaking. In some cases vasodepressor syncope may occur in which there is a fall in arterial pressure, a slowing of the pulse rate, but only a slight decrease in cardiac output. Since glucagon is known to markedly increase the blood flow of the splanchnic circulation, it may add to the constellation of symptoms. There is associated yawning and sighing, leading to frank hyperventilation, accompanied by pupillary dilatation and blurring of vision which precede loss of hearing. If the patient is seated or upright, the combination of hypotension and bradycardia causes cerebral blood flow to decrease leading to fleeting CNS effects such as nervousness, tremors, disorientation and syncope. Older patients, those worried about their condition, and those with markedly labile nervous systems may have a greater tendency to such reactions. Vasodepressor syncope usually clears promptly when the patient lies down.

The patient under discussion may indeed have had low-flow syndrome due to diarrhoea, to vasodepressor syncope, or to both. Considering the large number of patients who have received glucagon, this occurrence is extremely rare. However, the course of the events described also indicates that in all cases, particularly in the elderly patients, the referring physician and the radiologist should realize that no procedure is innocuous and that they must be sure that there is a good reason for doing the examination.

BIO-AVAILABILITY AND SAFETY

In studies of bio-availability and safety 2 mg glucagon and placebo have been given intramuscularly to 20 volunteer men every other day in a cross-over study. Following the administration of this dose of glucagon there was an increase in the fasting blood sugar, plasma glucagon, plasma insulin and no change in the plasma growth hormone levels during the period of the study[12]. There was a slight increase in the urinary output of norepinephrine, but this was not considered to be clinically or physiologically significant, especially as there was no change in the pulse rate or blood pressure in any of the volunteers.

There were no changes in the SMA 12/60, serum sodium, chloride, bicarbonate, urine analysis, RBC count, haematocrit, platelet count nor in the reticulocyte count. There was a slight increase in the WBC count, percent neutrophiles, and bands, and a decrease in the percent lymphocytes and serum potassium level. The results of the WBC and differential suggested that glucagon possesses the characteristics of one of the stress hormones[13]. This confirmed the opinions of Bloom et al.[14,15] and of Reynolds[16].

EFFECT ON POTASSIUM EXCRETION

After the administration of large doses of glucagon the serum potassium concentration may decrease. Vander Ark and Reynolds[17] reported that in four patients given large doses of glucagon the serum potassium concentration decreased from 4.5 to 3.2 mEq/l. This did not occur in 14 patients given glucagon and 20 mEq/l of potassium chloride. Following the administration of glucagon there is a release of potassium from the liver which produces a marked but transient hyperkalaemia. Mild but prolonged hypokalaemia is probably due to increased potassium excretion and increased uptake by tissues secondary to glucagon-induced insulin release. When a single dose of 2 mg glucagon was given intramuscularly Chernish et al.[12] saw a slight decrease in the plasma potassium after one hour (from 4.4 to 4.1 mEq/l). However, both values were within normal limits and not found to be statistically or considered to be clinically significant.

Parmley et al.[18] first reported that following the administration of glucagon there was a definite inotropic and chronotropic effect on the heart. The inotropic effect following glucagon administration occurred without increased ventricular irritability and was effective even in patients who were maximally digitalized. In other studies glucagon has been found to dilate the coronary vessels and the systemic arterioles, thus decreasing vascular resistance and increasing blood flow.

These reports suggested that glucagon may be of value in the treatment of certain cardiac conditions. Tinimis *et al.*[19] gave glucagon to cardiac patients in doses of 0.5 to 16 mg/h by continuous infusion for 5 to 166 hours. The total doses of glucagon given ranged from 25 to 996 mg per patient. One twenty-one-month old baby received approximately 8.25 mg in 165 hours. Patients from 1.8 to 78 years of age have been given glucagon for chronic congestive failure, post-perfusion low flow, and cardiogenic shock. Supplemental potassium was given to all of these patients in order to maintain the potassium balance. Loss of potassium following glucagon administration has been discussed in an earlier paragraph. Side effects of these doses of glucagon consisted primarily of nausea and vomiting. Lucchesi and Stutz[20] have written an excellent review of the use of glucagon in cardiac patients. Since new and more potent agents have been developed, the use of glucagon in patients with cardiac problems has been discontinued. However, the results of these studies indicate that large doses of glucagon may be given to patients with relative safety.

SENSITIVITY TO GLUCAGON

Glucagon is a straight chain polypeptide hormone unrelated to insulin. It is a much smaller molecule than insulin and it is extremely difficult to produce a high titre of antibodies to glucagon[21]. The glucagon that is manufactured from porcine and bovine pancreases has exactly the same amino acid sequence as human glucagon. Thus, it is apparently not recognized as a foreign protein. Because of these properties glucagon is a very poor antigen for man. Bloom[22] has stated that there appears to be a clear-cut hierarchy of immunogenicity among gut hormones. Secretin has been reported to be the most immunogenic, followed by gastric inhibitory peptide (GIP), and motilin. Vasoactive intestinal polypeptide (VIP) and glucagon are poor immunogens, and it is extremely difficult to obtain antiserum to pancreozymin.

In the 21 years that glucagon has been on the market millions of doses have been given. Over a period of approximately 4 years, cardiac patients received massive doses of glucagon by continuous intravenous infusion for many days. There appear, nevertheless, to be only five reports of possible sensitivity to glucagon, and all were related to very high doses. One patient developed a generalized erythematous rash, one a mild anaphylactoid type reaction with periorbital and perioral oedema, one developed a skin rash[23], one was described as having what was considered to be erythema multiforme[24], and one developed a hypotensive reaction[25].

There have been two reports of patients possibly being sensitive to trace amounts of insulin present in ampoules of glucagon[26, 27]. In connection with these two reports, glucagon has been given to patients allergic to insulin prior to insulin desensitization; these studies have failed to demonstrate a significant risk of allergic reaction to any insulin which might be present in commercial glucagon (Galloway, personal communication).

STIMULATION OF CATECHOLAMINES AND INSULIN

In 1960 Scian *et al.*[28] reported that there was a dose related increase in catecholamine excretion when glucagon was administered to dogs. Lawrence and Forland[29] suggested that glucagon may be useful as a provocative test for phaeochromocytoma. A follow-up of this suggestion indicated that glucagon may indeed be useful in diagnosis when phaeochromocytoma[28-39] and/or insulinoma[33-35, 40-42] are suspected of being present. When glucagon is given to a patient who has an insulinoma, large quantities of insulin may be released from the tumour. The patient may thus have an elevated blood glucose from the initial dose of glucagon followed by a marked drop in the blood glucose and develop symptoms of hypoglycaemia because of the release of insulin from the tumour. Thus far there have been three reports of patients with phaeochromocytoma having received glucagon inadvertently[36-38]

Glucagon given to a patient with phaeochromocytoma may stimulate the tumour to release large quantities of catecholamines with a consequent marked increase in blood pressure. Should this occur phentolamine mesefate given intravenously may well be tried in an attempt to control the blood pressure.

GLUCAGON AND THE DIABETIC PATIENT

Glucagon was initially marketed for use by diabetic patients for the treatment of hypoglycaemic reactions. Most diabetic patients carry sugar with them to take when they feel a hypoglycaemic reaction approaching. In instances when the patient does not get adequate warning, does not have sugar with him, or is asleep, when hypoglycaemia develops, glucagon may indeed be useful. The unconscious hypoglycaemic patient is, of course, unable to drink a sugar solution. Hypoglycaemic patients given 1 mg glucagon subcutaneously, intramuscularly, or intravenously, will release an adequate amount of glucose from the liver to abort the reaction. When the patient is able, a glass of glucose solution given orally will adequately complete the treatment and help to replace the liver glycogen.

Unfortunately, a number of authors have recently mentioned that glucagon should not be given to a diabetic patient; particularly not to the labile or brittle diabetic[43-49]. In fact, from the initial information presented, the drug is most useful in the treatment of the brittle or labile diabetic. Like a normal person, the diabetic will have an increase in blood glucose following an injection of glucagon. However, glucagon has a half-life of approximately 10 minutes. Thus, the blood glucose will be back to normal in one hour or less in a normal person. It will take the blood glucose somewhat longer to return to pre-treatment levels in the diabetic patient, particularly in the insulin-dependent diabetic.

The patient who has a seriously elevated blood glucose with hyperosmotic hyperglycaemia, or has hyperglycaemia and acidosis, has no reason to be in the radiology department for hypotonic studies. These patients are critically ill and need to have their diabetes brought under control before any such diagnostic studies are performed. One cannot believe that a radiologist would accept a patient for hypotonic diagnostic studies who may be partially or completely comatose.

Patients who are comatose may be brought to the radiology department because of a head injury. In such patients a CT scan of the head may be requested. However, we cannot see any reason for giving glucagon to a patient for a head scan. Patients with any injury to the liver or to the spleen may need an upper abdominal scan, but these patients are usually alert unless in shock due to blood loss. If there is any question concerning the patient's mental status blood glucose levels can rapidly be checked.

Although it is not the wisest course of action, we doubt that any harm will be done by giving one dose of glucagon to a patient with hyperglycaemia in acidosis. Many a brittle diabetic has received 1 mg glucagon when found unconscious. If he does not respond he is promptly taken to a hospital emergency room. If he was unconscious and hypoglycaemic it is possible that brain damage was prevented by the treatment with glucagon. If he was hyperglycaemic and acidotic, no harm was done.

Thus glucagon is a safe and effective drug to produce hypotonia of the gastrointestinal tract and the diabetic patient should not be deprived of this excellent diagnostic procedure.

SUMMARY AND CONCLUSIONS

Glucagon has been reported to have few and minimal side effects in doses of 0.025 to 2 mg. Reports of side effects at a dose of 0.1 mg of glucagon given intravenously have not been greater than those reported for placebo. It does not have the contraindications to its use that anticholingergic drugs have.

Since it is a protein, allergic reactions are possible, but during the 21 years of its use there have been extremely few reports of adverse reactions. For diagnostic radiographic or CT scan of the abdomen patients with suspected, or with a history of, phaeochromocytoma and/or insulinoma should not receive glucagon, but these are very rare conditions.

Following the administration of glucagon to normal people there is an increase in the serum glucose, insulin and glucagon levels. There appear to be no changes in blood chemistry, except for a slight decrease in serum potassium. Studies have shown there to be no changes in urine analysis, red blood count, haematocrit, platelet count or reticulocyte count; there is a slight increase in the white blood count, percent neutrophiles and bands, and a decrease in the percent lymphocytes.

These results indicate that glucagon is a safe and effective drug to produce hypotonia of the gastrointestinal tract. Reports of side effects have been few and minimal, and have consisted mainly of nausea and/or vomiting.

References

1. Miller, R. E., Chernish, S. M. and Brunelle, R. L. (1979). Gastrointestinal radiography with glucagon. *Gastrointest. Radiol.*, **4**, 1
2. Levenstein, S. (1981). Glucagon, diarrhea, and cerebral symptoms. (Letter to the editor) *J. Am. Med. Assoc.*, **246**, 1545
3. Miller, R. E., Chernish, S. M., Brunelle, R. L. and Rosenak, B. D. (1978). Double blind radiographic study of dose response to intravenous glucagon for hypotonic duodenography. *Radiology*, **127**, 55
4. Barbezat, G. O. and Grossman, M. I. (1971). Cholera-like diarrhoea induced by glucagon plus gastrin. *Lancet*, **1**, 1025
5. Barbezat, G. O. and Grossman, M. I. (1971). Effect of glucagon on water and electrolyte movement in jejunum and ileum of dog. *Gastroenterology*, **60**, 762
6. Barbezat, G. O. and Grossman, M. I. (1971). Intestinal secretion. Stimulation by peptides. *Science*, **174**, 422
7. Hicks, T. and Turnberg, L. A. (1974). Influence of glucagon on the human jejunum. *Gastroenterology*, **67**, 1114
8. Mallinson, C. M., Bloom, S. R., Warin, A. P., Salmon, P. R. and Cox, B. (1974). A glucagonoma syndrome. *Lancet*, **2**, 1
9. Schlaeger, R. (1967). Examination of the small intestine. In Margulis, A. and Burhenne, H. J. (eds.) *Alimentary Tract Roentgenology*, Vol. II, chapter 22, pp. 591–592. (Saint Louis: C. V. Mosby)
10. Weintraub, S. and Williams, R. G. (1949). A rapid method of roentgenologic examination of the small intestine. *Am. J. Roentgenol.*, **61**, 45
11. Weissler, A. M. and Warren, J. V. (1959). Vasodepressor syncope. Review. *Am. Heart J.*, **57**, 786
12. Chernish, S. M., Davidson, J. A., Brunelle, R. L., Miller, R. E. and Rosenak, B. D. (1975). Response of normal subjects to a single 2-milligram dose of glucagon administered intramuscularly. *Arch. Int. Pharmacodyn.*, **218**, 312

13. Wintrobe, M. D. (1967). *Clinical Hematology*, edition 6, p. 262. (Philadelphia: Lea and Febiger)
14. Bloom, S. R. (1973). Glucagon, a stress hormone. *Postgrad. Med. J.*, **49**, 607
15. Bloom, S. R., Daniel, P. M., Johnston, D. E., Ogawa, O. and Pratt, O. E. (1973). Release of glucagon induced by stress. *Q. J. Exp. Physiol.*, **58**, 99
16. Reynolds, A. E. (1971). The beta cell and its responses. Summarizing remarks and some contributions from Geneva. *Diabetes*, **21** (suppl.), 619
17. Vander Ark, C. R. and Reynolds, E. W. (1970). Clinical evaluation of glucagon by continuous infusion in the treatment of low cardiac output states. *Am. Heart J.*, **79**, 481
18. Parmley, W. W., Glick, G. and Sonnenbleck, E. H. (1968). Cardiovascular effects of glucagon in man. *N. Engl. J. Med.*, **279**, 12
19. Tinimis, G. C., Lin, R., Ramos, R. G. and Gordon, S. (1973). Prolonged glucagon infusion in cardiac failure. *J. Am. Med. Assoc.*, **223**, 293
20. Lucchesi, B. R. and Stutz, D. R. (1970). The cardiovascular pharmacology and potential clinical uses of glucagon. *Univ. Mich. Med. Cent. J.*, **36**, 101
21. Unger, R. H. (1975). Action of glucagon as adjunct to gastrointestinal X-ray film examination. (Letter to the editor) *J. Am. Med. Assoc.*, **231**, 80
22. Bloom, S. R. (1974). Hormones of the gastrointestinal tract. *Br. Med. Bull.*, **30**, 62
23. Barber, S. G. and Hammer, J. D. (1976). Skin rash in patients receiving glucagon. (Letter to the editor) *Lancet*, **2**, 1138
24. Edel, S. L. (1980). Erythema multiforme secondary to intravenous glucagon. *Am. J. Roentgenol.*, **134**, 385
25. Carleton, J. L., Greben, S. E. and Schulman, J. L. (1957). Hypotensive reaction following the use of glucagon. *Arch. Intern. Med.*, **99**, 817
26. Thorell, J. I. and Persson, B. (1970). Side effects of insulin contaminating commercial glucagon. (Letter to the editor) *Lancet*, **2**, 52
27. Kitabchi, A. E., Lamkin, N., Jr., Lieberman, P., Ayyagari, V. and Baskin, F. K. (1975). Allergic response to glucagon injection as a result of insulin contamination. *J. Clin. Endocrinol. Metab.*, **41**, 863
28. Scian, L. F., Westermann, C. D. and Verdesca, A. S. (1960). Adrenocortical and medullary effects of glucagon. *Am. J. Physiol.*, **199**, 867
29. Lawrence, A. M. and Forland, M. G. (1964). Glucagon: provocative tests for pheochromocytoma. *J. Lab. Clin. Med.*, **64**, 878 (Abstract)
30. Lawrence, A. M. (1965). A new provocative test for pheochromocytoma. *Ann. Intern. Med.*, **63**, 905 (Abstract)
31. Lawrence, A. M. (1967). Glucagon provocative test for pheochromocytoma. *Ann. Intern. Med.*, **66**, 1091
32. Sheps, S. G. and Maher, F. T. (1968). Histamine and glucagon tests in diagnosis of pheochromocytoma. *J. Am. Med. Assoc.*, **205**, 895
33. Lefèbvre, P. J. and Unger, R. H. (1972). *Glucagon: Molecular Physiology, Clinical and Therapeutic Implications*, pp. 299–318 (Oxford: Pergamon)
34. Lawrence, A. M. (1969). Glucagon. *Ann. Rev. Med.*, **30**, 207
35. Lawrence, A. M. (1970). Glucagon in medicine. New ideas for an old hormone. *Med. Clin. N. Am.*, **54**, 183
36. Biggs, I. (1978). Pheochromocytoma diagnosed during barium meal. *Br. J. Radiol.*, **51**, 981
37. Geelhoed, G. W. (1980). CAT scans and catecholamines. *Surgery*, **87**, 719
38. McLoughlin, M. J., Langer, B. and Wilson, D. R. (1981). Life-threatening reaction to glucagon in a patient with pheochromocytoma. (Letter to the editor) *Radiology*, **140**, 841
39. Cremer, G. M., Molnar, G. D., Moxness, K. E., Sheps, S. G., Maker, F. T. and Jones, J. D. (1963). Hormonal and biochemical response to glucagon administration in patients with pheochromocytoma and in control subjects. *Mayo Clin. Proc.*, **43**, 161

40. Marks, V. and Samols, E. (1968). Glucagon test for insulinoma. A chemical study in 25 cases. *J. Clin. Path.*, **21**, 346
41. Ahneda, A., Maruhama, Y., Itabashi, H., Horigome, K., Yanbe, A., Ishii, S., Masamichi, C., Kai, Y., Abe, R. and Yamagata, S. (1975). Diagnostic value of intravenous glucagon test in insulinoma. *Tohuku J. Exp. Med.*, **116**, 205
42. Kumar, D., Mektalia, S. D. and Miller, L. V. (1974). Diagnostic use of glucagon-induced insulin response. Studies in patients with insulinoma or other hypoglycemic conditions. *Ann. Intern. Med.*, **80**, 697
43. Simpkins, K. C. (1976). Radiology now. The colon pacified. *Br. J. Radiol.*, **49**, 303
44. Jerele, J. J. (1976). Use of glucagon as the hypotonic agent in barium enema examination. *J. Am. Osteopath. Assoc.*, **76**, 264
45. Laufer, I. (1979). *Double Contract Gastrointestinal Radiology with Endoscopic Correlation*, p. 63. (Philadelphia: W. B. Saunders)
46. Ferrucci, J. T. (1974). Hypotonic duodenography. In *Syllabus, Categorical Course on Radiology of Gastrointestinal Tract Disease*, pp. 2 and 11. (Chicago: Radiological Society of North America)
47. Paul, F. and Freyschmidt, J. (1976). Anwendung von Glukagon bei endoskopischen und röntgenologischen Untersuchungen des Gastrointestinaltrakts. *Fortschr. Röntgenstr.*, **125**, 31
48. Op Den Orth, J. (1979). *The Standard Biphasic Contrast Examination of the Stomach and Duodenum*, p. 10. (Boston: Martinus Nijhoff)
49. Evans, A. F. and Whitehouse, G. H. (1979). The effect of glucagon on infusion cholangiography. *Clin. Radiol.*, **30**, 499

Address for correspondence

Professor R. E. Miller
Indiana University Medical Center
Department of Radiology
1100 West Michigan Street
Indianapolis, IN 46223, USA

5

The possible physiological role of glucagon on gastro-esophageal function

J. CHRISTIANSEN

Glucagon inhibits gastric secretion as well as gastro-esophageal motor function in man. There is evidence that some of these inhibitory effects of glucagon may be of physiological relevance.

GASTRIC SECRETION

Exogenous administration of glucagon in pharmacological doses inhibits basal, meal- and pentagastrin-stimulated gastric acid secretion[1-4], whereas there is conflicting evidence as to the effect on histamine-induced acid secretion[5, 6]. These observations have given rise to a series of studies on the possible role of glucagon in the physiological inhibition of gastric acid secretion.

Maximal pentagastrin-stimulated acid secretion is inhibited by approximately 80% after a bolus injection of 4 mg glucagon[1]. To study physiological interactions, however, it is necessary to use submaximal doses of pentagastrin, preferably doses in the range of D_{50} for the subjects under study, and doses of glucagon which result in plasma concentrations comparable to those seen after a meal.

Plasma glucagon concentrations can be determined by a highly specific radioimmunoassay. Fasting levels of glucagon are about 10–20 pmol/l with an increase[7] after a protein-rich meal to about 60–80 pmol/l.

Figure 1 shows the effect of increasing doses of glucagon on acid secretion stimulated by pentagastrin $130 \, \text{ng} \, \text{kg}^{-1} \, \text{h}^{-1}$, which was the mean D_{50} for the healthy subjects studied[2]. The dose-dependent effect of glucagon is obvious, and a dose of $16 \, \mu\text{g} \, \text{kg}^{-1} \, \text{h}^{-1}$ almost completely blocks the acid response. A dose of glucagon of $300 \, \text{ng} \, \text{kg}^{-1} \, \text{h}^{-1}$ results in plasma glucagon concentrations[8] of 60–80 pmol/l, and thus seems to be an adequate dose to use in physiological studies.

Appraisal of the possible role of glucagon in the physiological inhibition of gastric acid secretion requires knowledge of the effect of the hormone on meal-stimulated acid secretion when administered or released in concentrations similar to those seen after a meal. Figure 2 shows the results of a study in which exogenous glucagon was administered in a dose of $300 \, \text{ng} \, \text{kg}^{-1} \, \text{h}^{-1}$ and endogenous glucagon released by the intravenous infusion of *l*-arginine in a dose of $0.6 \, \text{g} \, \text{kg}^{-1} \, \text{h}^{-1}$. Compared to the control experiment (NaCl) glucagon as well as arginine significantly reduced the meal-stimulated acid response as determined by intragastric titration[8]. The plasma concentrations of glucagon obtained during infusion of glucagon and *l*-arginine were almost identical and similar to those seen after a protein-rich meal (Figure 3). The fact that meal-induced glucagon concentrations in the control study amounted to only about

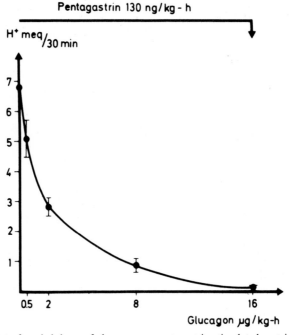

Figure 1 Effect of graded doses of glucagon on pentagastrin-stimulated gastric acid output

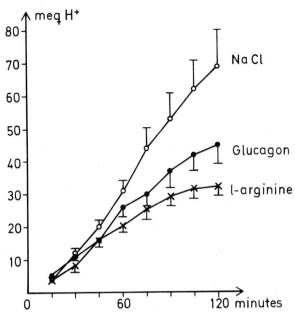

Figure 2 Cumulated meal-stimulated gastric acid secretion during intravenous infusion of saline, glucagon and *l*-arginine. Mean ±SEM

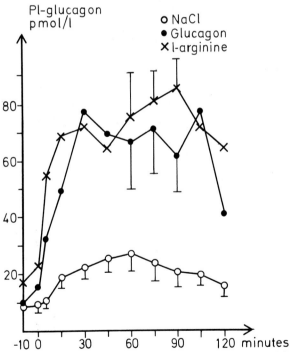

Figure 3 Plasma glucagon concentrations during intragastric titration and infusion of saline, glucagon and *l*-arginine. Mean ± SEM

one-third of those seen during the infusion of glucagon and *l*-arginine is due to the intragastric titration technique, which profoundly interferes with gastric emptying. When the stomach is allowed to empty the meal in a normal fashion, plasma concentrations of the same order of magnitude are found.

Although the same plasma glucagon levels were obtained with infusion of glucagon and *l*-arginine the latter was found to be a more potent inhibitor of acid secretion. This was not due to differences in gastrin release (Figure 4), or different blood glucose levels (Figure 5). *l*-Arginine may, however, release hormones or peptides other than glucagon and does in fact release growth hormone. Since the release of this hormone is delayed compared to glucagon[9] it is most unlikely that it is this which is responsible for the pronounced acid inhibition appearing early during infusion of *l*-arginine. Consequently, certain important necessary conditions for establishing a physiological role of glucagon as an inhibitor of acid secretion are fulfilled: gastrin- and meal-stimulated acid secretion are inhibited in doses of the hormone resulting in plasma concentrations equal to those seen after a meal, and endogenous release of the hormone in the same concentrations has the same effect.

Since defects in acid inhibitory mechanisms may be a pathogenetic factor in duodenal ulcer disease, glucagon mediated acid inhibition was compared in

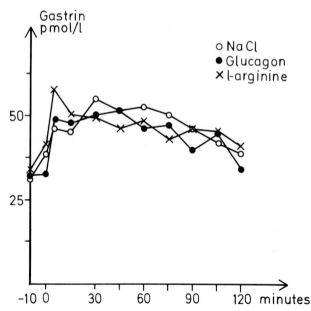

Figure 4 Mean serum gastrin concentrations during intragastric titration and infusion of saline, glucagon and *l*-arginine

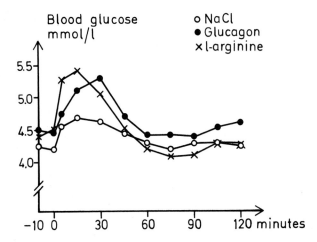

Figure 5 Blood glucose concentrations during intravenous infusion of saline, glucagon and *l*-arginine

healthy subjects and in duodenal ulcer patients. Endogenously released glucagon (Figure 6) as well as exogenously administered glucagon in a dose of $300 \, ng \, kg^{-1} \, h^{-1}$ showed exactly the same degree of inhibition in the two groups, suggesting that duodenal ulcer patients do not have any defect in glucagon mediated inhibition of gastric acid secretion[10].

The mechanisms of acid inhibition by glucagon are still obscure. It has been demonstrated that the interaction of glucagon and gastrin follows non-competitive kinetics[2], which is also to be expected when the structure–activity relationship is taken into consideration. In agreement with this concept, no augmentation of acid inhibition was found when glucagon and cholecysto-kinin were administered simultaneously on a background infusion of pentagastrin[11]. Furthermore, recent studies have shown that intact vagal innervation of the fundic gland area is a prerequisite of acid inhibition by glucagon since glucagon induced inhibition of pentagastrin stimulated acid secretion was completely abolished by parietal cell vagotomy[12,13]. This is true whether glucagon is released endogenously or administered exogenously (Figure 7). The nature of this vagus–glucagon interaction is unknown, but as a first step to elucidate this observation further studies on the acid inhibitory effect of glucagon during cholinergic and adrenergic blockade are in progress.

Glucagon increases the negativity of gastric mucosal potential difference (PD) in man[14] coinciding in time with the acid inhibitory effect[15]. Gastric

73

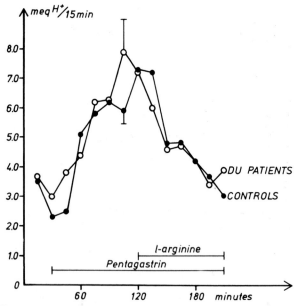

Figure 6 Effect of arginine infusion on pentagastrin-stimulated gastric acid secretion in duodenal ulcer (DU) patients and normal subjects. Mean $\pm$ SEM

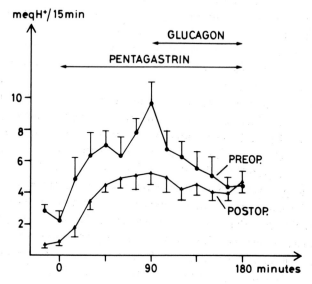

Figure 7 Effect of glucagon infusion $(300\,ng\,kg^{-1}\,h^{-1})$ on pentagastrin-stimulated $(100\,ng\,kg^{-1}\,h^{-1})$ acid secretion in duodenal ulcer patients before and after parietal cell vagotomy

biopsies show that the acid inhibition and increased negative PD are associated with a significant reduction in secretory canalicular membrane area[15], findings which have previously been linked to the increase in PD caused by acid inhibitors[16].

Data on the effect of glucagon on pepsin secretion are limited compared to data on acid secretion. Bolus injection of pharmacological doses of glucagon had no effect on unstimulated pepsin secretion[17], whereas histamine stimulated secretion was significantly inhibited[18]. In a recent study on interaction of pentagastrin and glucagon in physiological doses, it was found that glucagon reduced the pepsin secretory potency of pentagastrin[19]. This is in contrast to the structurally similar secretin which stimulates pepsin secretion.

GASTRO-ESOPHAGEAL MOTILITY

Gastrointestinal hormones control motility by modulation of gastrointestinal pace-setter potentials, i.e., by modifying frequency, amplitude and duration of action-potentials[20]. Glucagon inhibits proximal[20,21] and distal gastric[21] contractions probably resulting in a reduced gastric emptying rate[20]. The physiological significance of these observations is unknown.

Glucagon inhibits lower esophageal sphincter (LES) pressure, and its pharmacological effect in patients suffering from achalasia and esophageal food obstruction is well documented[22,23]. Whether the action of glucagon on LES pressure has any physiological significance is, however, doubtful.

Only supraphysiological doses of glucagon affect resting LES pressure[24] and the effect of smaller doses of glucagon on pentagastrin stimulated LES pressure has only been demonstrated after pulse injection[24]. Furthermore, the interpretation of these findings is complicated by evidence suggesting that gastrin has no physiological effect on LES pressure[24,25]. Endogenously released glucagon has no effect on resting LES pressure[26] whereas pentagastrin stimulated LES pressure has been shown to be inhibited to approximately the same degree as after infusion of $1.6 \mu g \, kg^{-1} \, h^{-1}$ of glucagon (Figure 8), although the latter resulted in a markedly higher plasma glucagon concentration[27] (Figure 9), suggesting that infusion of arginine has an effect on pentagastrin stimulated LES pressure unrelated to glucagon release. The kinetics of interaction with pentagastrin on LES pressure is of the mixed type[26] and there is no interaction with the structurally similar secretin[28].

The mechanism of action of glucagon on LES pressure is unknown, but studies on the feline LES suggest that glucagon acts at the preganglionic level of the sympathetic pathway within the adrenal glands[29].

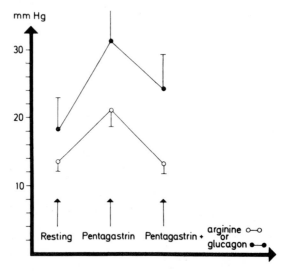

Figure 8 Lower esophageal sphincter pressure during infusion of pentagastrin $0.5 \mu g\,kg^{-1}\,h^{-1}$, pentagastrin + glucagon $1.6\,\mu g\,kg^{-1}\,h^{-1}$, pentagastrin + l-arginine $0.6\,g\,kg^{-1}\,h^{-1}$

At present there is no evidence of a physiological action of glucagon on the LES, and in doses which reduce LES pressure glucagon does not affect esophageal peristalsis[24].

In conclusion, there is strong evidence that pancreatic glucagon is a physiological inhibitor of gastric secretion and that the acid inhibitory effect seems to be identical in healthy individuals and in duodenal ulcer patients. In contrast, glucagon is unlikely to exert any physiological effect on the lower esophageal sphincter. The mechanism of action is unknown, but intact vagal innervation of the fundic gland area is necessary for the acid inhibitory effect and there is evidence that the effect on the lower esophageal sphincter is mediated through the sympathetic nervous system.

References

1. Christiansen, J. and Hendel, L. (1973). The effect of glucagon in pentagastrin-induced gastric acid secretion and serum calcium concentration in man. *Scand. J. Gastroenterol.*, **8**, 81
2. Christiansen, J., Holst, J. J. and Kalaja, E. (1976). Inhibition of gastric acid secretion in man by exogenous and endogenous pancreatic glucagon. *Gastroenterology*, **70**, 688
3. Dotevall, G., Kock, N. G. and Walan, A. (1969). Inhibition of pentagastrin-induced gastric acid secretion in man given intravenously. *Scand. J. Gastroenterol.*, **4**, 713

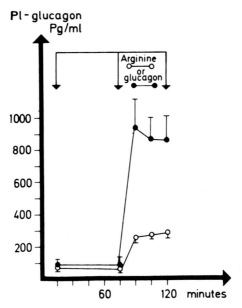

Figure 9 Plasma glucagon concentrations during infusion of glucagon $1.6\,\mu g\,kg^{-1}\,h^{-1}$ and during infusion of l-arginine $0.6\,g\,kg^{-1}\,h^{-1}$

4. Christiansen, J. and Hendel, L. (1974). The effect of glucagon on pentagastrin-induced gastric secretion of sodium, potassium and calcium in man. *Scand. J. Gastroenterol.*, **9**, 437

5. Melrose, A. G. (1960). Effect of glucagon on gastric secretion in man. *Gut*, **1**, 142

6. Cohen, W., Mazure, P., Dreiling, D. and Janowitz, H. D. (1960). The effect of glucagon on histamin-stimulated gastric secretion in man. *Gastroenterology*, **39**, 48

7. Rehfeld, J. F., Holst, J. J. and Kühl, L. (1978). The effect of gastrin on basal and aminoacid-stimulated insulin and glucagon secretion in man. *Eur. J. Clin. Invest.*, **8**, 5

8. Loud, F. B., Froberg, D., Reichardt, J., Holst, J. J., Rehfeld, J. F. and Christiansen, J. (1978). Inhibition of meal-stimulated gastric acid secretion in man by exogenous and endogenous pancreatic glucagon. *Scand. J. Gastroenterol.*, **13**, 795

9. Merimell, T. J., Lillicrap, D. A. and Rabino-Witz, D. (1965). Effect of arginine on serum levels of human growth hormone. *Lancet*, **2**, 668

10. Loud, F. B., Kirkegaard, P., Holst, J. J. and Christiansen, J. (1980). Effect of endogenous pancreatic glucagon in duodenal ulcer patients and normal subjects. *Scand. J. Gastroenterol.*, **15**, 711

11. Hendel, L., Jørgensen, S. P., Christiansen, J. and Henriksen, F. W. (1976). Combined effect of glucagon and cholecystokinin on gastric secretion in man. *Scand. J. Gastroenterol.* (Suppl.), **37**, 43

12. Loud, F. B., Christiansen, J., Holst, J. J., Petersen, B. and Kirkegaard, P. (1981). Effect of endogenous pancreatic glucagon on gastric acid secretion in patients with duodenal ulcer before and after parietal cell vagotomy. *Gut*, **22**, 359

13. Olsen, P. S., Kirkegaard, P., Holst, J. J. and Christiansen, J. (1981). Vagal control of glucagon induced inhibition of gastric acid secretion in duodenal ulcer patients. *Scand. J. Gastroenterol.* (In press)
14. Tarnawski, A., Krause, W. J. and Ivey, K. J. (1978). Effect of glucagon on aspirin-induced gastric mucosal damage in man. *Gastroenterology*, **74**, 240
15. Ivey, K. J., Tarnawski, A., Sherman, D., Krause, W. J., Ackman, K., Burks, M. and Hewett, J. (1980). Quantitative ultrastructural analysis of the human parietal cell during acid inhibition and increase of gastric potential difference by glucagon. *Gut*, **21**, 3
16. Forte, T. M., Machen, T. E. and Fork, J. G. (1977). Ultrastructural changes in oxyntic cells associated with secretory function: a membrane recycling hypothesis. *Gastroenterology*, **73**, 941
17. Brooks, A. M. and Grossman, M. I. (1970). Effect of secretin and cholecystokinin on pentagastrin-stimulated gastric secretion in man. *Gastroenterology*, **59**, 114
18. Cohen, M., Mazure, P., Dreiling, D. A. and Janowitz, H. D. (1960). Effect of glucagon on histamin-stimulated gastric secretion in man. *Gastroenterology*, **39**, 48
19. Christiansen, J., Holst, J. J. and Molin, J. (1981). Interaction of glucagon and pentagastrin on pepsin secretion in healthy subjects. *Gut*. (In press)
20. Thomas, P. A., Akwari, O. E. and Kelly, K. A. (1979). Hormonal control of gastrointestinal motility. *Wld. J. Surg.*, **3**, 545
21. Rees, W. D. W., Miller, L. J. and Malagelada, J.-R. (1980). Dyspepsia, antral motor dysfunction and gastric stasis of solids. *Gastroenterology*, **78**, 360
22. Jennewein, H. M., Waldeck, F., Siewert, R., Weiser, F. and Thimm, R. (1973). The interaction of glucagon and pentagastrin on the lower esophageal sphincter in man and dog. *Gut*, **14**, 861
23. Pillari, G., Bank, S., Kutzka, I. and Fulco, J. D. (1979). Meat bolus impaction of the lower esophagus associated with a paraesophageal hernia. *Am. J. Gastroenterol.*, **71**, 287
24. Hogan, W. J., Dodds, W. J., Hoke, S. E., Reid, D. P., Kalkhoff, R. K. and Arndorfer, R. C. (1975). Effect of glucagon on esophageal motor function. *Gastroenterology*, **69**, 160
25. Goyal, R. K. and McGuigan, J. E. (1976). Is gastrin a major determinant of basal lower esophageal sphincter pressure? *J. Clin. Invest.*, **57**, 291
26. Jaffer, S. S., Makhlouf, G. M., Schorr, B. A. and Zfass, A. M. (1974). Nature and kinetics of inhibition of lower esophageal sphincter pressure by glucagon. *Gastroenterology*, **67**, 42
27. Christiansen, J., Lauritzen, K., Moesgaard, J. and Holst, J. J. (1977). Effect of endogenous and exogenous glucagon on pentagastrin-stimulated lower esophageal sphincter pressure in man. *Scand. J. Gastroenterol.*, **12**, 33
28. Christiansen, J. and Borgeskov, S. (1974). The effect of glucagon and the combined effect of glucagon and secretin on lower esophageal sphincter pressure in man. *Scand. J. Gastroenterol.*, **9**, 615
29. Behar, J., Field, S. and Marin, C. (1979). Effect of glucagon, secretin and vasoactive intestinal polypeptide on the feline lower esophageal sphincter: mechanisms of action. *Gastroenterology*, **77**, 1001

Address for correspondence

Dr. J. Christiansen,
Køvenhavns Amts Sygehus,
Kirurgisk Afdeling D,
DK-2600 Glostrup,
Denmark.

DISCUSSION

Oriol Bosch: You said that you saw no effects on somatostatin release. How did you measure somatostatin? Was it a simple radioimmunoassay in blood? If so, I have my doubts about the real value of your results. When one does a chromatographic run one finds at least three different specimens of somatostatin activity in plasma, and I do not think it does any good to measure those levels of radioimmunoassay activity in plasma when we do not know what the biological meaning of each peak of activity is.

Christiansen: Well, I cannot argue with you since I am not the radioimmunologist in our team. Our radioimmunoasay is based on rabbit antibodies.

Vilardell: The vagotomy you were talking about, is that parietal cell vagotomy?

Christiansen: Yes Dr. Bloom, from London, showed that release of glucagon, after a protein rich meal, was significantly reduced after truncal vagotomy, but not affected by selective vagotomy. Selective vagotomy showed the same response as in normal persons (Bloom, S. R. *et al.* (1974). *Lancet,* **2,** 546). In our subjects the release was the same as in normal subjects, so it is in the target cells that something happens. But I am afraid I cannot say which mechanism is responsible for this.

Vilardell: Was there any effect on gastric distension?

Christiansen: I do not know.

Miller: I understand that there is no normal physiological effect of glucagon except on the lower esophageal sphincter, but are you saying that there is no relaxation of the lower esophageal sphincter at pharmacological doses such as 1 or 2 mg?

Christiansen: No, I did not say that. Hogan and co-workers showed that at a dose of 1 μg/kg – which gives plasma concentrations above physiological levels – it has no effect, contrary to higher doses, I think 10 μg/kg (Hogan, W. J. *et al.* (1975). *Gastroenterology,* **69,** 160).

Jaspan: I think the observations about the physiologic control of gastric acid secretion are very important. I just want to add an extra caution, and that is that in general, after a meal, glucagon levels are not altered because most meals are a mixture of carbohydrates and protein. I agree with you that if a meal was a pure protein meal, which in fact very few of us eat, you would get the kind of levels that you showed, i.e., three- or four-fold elevated levels of glucagon. In a normal situation, however, when an 'average' mixed meal is taken, the levels are not much changed. If it is a high carbohydrate meal, the levels are suppressed. If it happens to be a predominantly protein meal, the levels would be elevated in proportion to the amount of protein taken, and that may have something to do with gastric acid release in response to different meals.

Christiansen: The meal we used for our study of plasma concentration is the same meal as we used for intragastric titration, i.e. a steak meal of a 300 g sirloin steak, with no potatoes.

Jaspan: That will certainly increase glucagon, three- or four-fold.

Diamant: I find it very interesting that you have demonstrated that vagotomy reverses the inhibitory effect of glucagon on gastric acid secretion. This agrees well with the experimental indications we have obtained on the inhibitory action of glucagon and glucagon-(1–21)-peptide on cholinergic transmission.

Christiansen: I certainly agree. This is something that we are anxious to explore further.

Skucas: Is it not true that after therapeutic doses of glucagon the blood flow through gastric mucosa decreases considerably, while that through the muscle areas increases considerably? If this is true, the gastric acid inhibition seen with glucagon could perhaps be due to the decreased blood flow rather than to anything else. Do you not think this so?

Christiansen: This subject has been studied by Ginsberg, B. *et al.* (1971) (*Gastroenterology*, **60**, 775). It seems, in fact, that the inhibition of gastric acid secretion must supersede the effect on blood flow. If one mimics the reduction in blood flow with other drugs, one does not find any inhibition of acid secretion. So I do think that there must be another mechanism or mechanisms involved.

6

The role of glucagon in the management of colonic disorders and colonic surgery

O. DANIEL

The ability of glucagon to inhibit intestinal spasm and motility and also to augment intestinal blood flow suggests the possibility of therapeutic use in a variety of conditions, only one of which has as yet been established by adequate controlled clinical trials.

The only therapeutic use of glucagon of value as proven by a clinical double-blind cross-over study is in the preparation of patients for barium enema examination[1]. In colonoscopy a small preliminary comparative test between glucagon and placebo showed that complete examination of the colon could be performed more speedily and with much less discomfort to the patient[2], but subsequent larger randomized double-blind studies of glucagon versus placebo showed that the administration of glucagon either made the procedure more difficult[3] or had no demonstrable effect[4].

The ability of glucagon to increase intestinal blood flow[5-7] suggests a possible use in various conditions marked by ischaemic changes or as an aid to restoration of circulation following reduction of strangulation but there are, as yet, no published reports of clinical trials.

The use of glucagon has been tried with encouraging clinical results, but its value not yet proven by controlled trials, in the following conditions.

THE USE OF GLUCAGON IN THE TREATMENT OF SYMPTOMS SUGGESTIVE OF ACUTE DIVERTICULITIS

The hypothesis that symptoms of acute diverticulitis are sometimes due only to spasm and hypermotility[8] in hypertrophied colonic muscle[9] suggested to Daniel et al.[10] that the ability of glucagon to reduce intestinal motility[11,12] might be of therapeutic use in this condition. Accordingly, over a two-year period ending in December 1973, twenty consecutive patients admitted as emergencies to one general surgical unit, with symptoms suggestive of acute diverticulitis, received intravenous injections of glucagon as primary treatment. The results were compared, retrospectively, with a matched group of fifteen patients who had received conventional treatment for similar symptoms during the preceding eighteen months.

In both groups of patients the clinical condition was characterized by abdominal pain with localized tender swelling of the iliac or pelvic colon. Bowel function was usually disturbed, either with constipation, diarrhoea, or, rarely, alternating constipation and diarrhoea. Many of the patients had pyrexia with leukocytosis, nausea, vomiting, abdominal distension, or passed mucus or blood per rectum. In both groups of patients the initial clinical diagnosis was later confirmed and the presence of other pathology excluded, as far as possible, by means of sigmoidoscopy and barium enema examination (Table 1).

Glucagon treatment

Crystalline glucagon was dissolved immediately before use in the accompanying diluent. In the first eight patients 10 ml of solution containing 1 mg glucagon was injected directly into a forearm vein over a period of 5–8 seconds. In the next six patients 1 mg glucagon was injected more slowly into a vein over 8–10 minutes. These injections were repeated at four-hourly intervals over 36 hours, a total of nine doses. The remaining six patients received 4.5 mg glucagon in 50 ml of diluent by continuous slow pump infusion over two consecutive periods of eighteen hours. Initially diet was restricted to fluids, gradually returning to normal as symptoms subsided, and then supplemented with 50 g unrefined bran daily. Four patients with signs suggestive of actual or impending pericolic abscess received, in addition, courses of ampicillin or tetracycline.

Table 1 Data relating to 35 study patients admitted to hospital suffering acute diverticulitis

(a) Group treated with glucagon

Patient	Sex	Age	Pain	Constipation	Diarrhoea	Vomiting	Nausea	Rectal discharge		Abdominal signs	Temp °C	Leukocyte count W.C.C./cm
								Mucus	Blood			
1	F	88	+		+		+			M	37.5	11 600
2	F	87	+		+	+		+		M	37.0	7 200
3	F	83	+					+		M	37.1	7 400
4	F	62	+	+A	+A	+		+		M	37.2	10 300
5	M	66	+	+						G	37.0	6 800
6	F	69	+	+		+				M D	37.0	9 500
7	F	73	+	+		+				G	37.5	9 100
8	F	60	+				+			M	37.0	12 500
9	F	74	+	+						M	38.0	10 700
10	M	55	+	+	+					M	38.2	5 600
11	F	41	+					+		M	38.0	5 700
12	M	65	+			+	+			M	37.0	8 000
13	F	31	+		+	+	+			M D	37.5	6 500
14	M	80	+		+	+				G D	37.0	8 200
15	F	84	+	+		+				G	37.5	9 500
16	F	77	+	+		+				G	37.0	20 200
17	F	58	+		+	+				G	36.5	15 100
18	F	73	+		+					M D	37.2	24 000
19	M	54	+	+						M D	38.0	14 000
20	M	75	+		+			+	+	G D	38.3	20 500

Table 1 (Continued)

(b) Control group

No.	Sex	Age									Temp.	
1	F	79	+	+			+		G	D	36.5	6 300
2	F	75	+	+		+	+	+	G	D	37.0	6 200
3	M	84	+	+					M		37.1	5 100
4	F	76	+	+A					M	D	37.0	13 000
5	F	62	+	+A	+	+			M		37.2	4 800
6	F	65	+	+	+	+			G		37.0	12 500
7	F	64	+	+	+				M	D	37.1	7 300
8	F	67	+			+			G		37.3	7 900
9	F	83	+	+	+	+			M	D	37.0	7 400
10	M	70	+	+	+	+			M		37.0	7 200
11	F	70	+	+	+				M		36.5	13 500
12	M	54	+		+	+			M		38.5	16 600
13	M	42	+	+	+			+	G	D	38.6	15 700
14	F	65	+	+	+				M		37.5	15 200
15	F	68	+		+				M		38.2	21 000

Abdominal signs:

M = tender mass in left iliac fossa or pelvis.

G = tenderness with guarding or rigidity in left iliac fossa.

D = abdominal distension.

+A = alternating constipation and diarrhoea

84

Conventional treatment

The fifteen patients chosen retrospectively as controls received paracetamol or pethidine in doses adequate to relieve pain, parenteral tetracycline or ampicillin if there was fever or other sign of inflammation, and naso-gastric suction and intravenous fluids when there were signs of obstruction or dehydration. The majority also received repeated intramuscular injections of 20 mg hyoscine butylbromide or 30 mg propantheline bromide for the relief of colonic muscle spasm. Initially, oral feeding was restricted to fluids but light diet was given as soon as it could be tolerated, and supplemented with 50 g unrefined bran daily.

Results of glucagon treatment

The administration of glucagon was followed within 6–24 hours (mean 12 hours) by virtually complete relief from the main symptoms and also by substantial improvement in general condition. The most constant and noticeable benefit was relief of pain which was always the predominant complaint on admission. No patient receiving glucagon needed analgesics, though these drugs are usually a necessary part of conventional treatment. The dull aching discomfort related to the swelling of the affected gut disappeared as quickly as did generalized abdominal pain. Disturbance of bowel function was corrected within an average of 12 hours. Patients who had suffered constipation which was resistant to all other treatment, including suppositories and enemas, were greatly relieved by effortless and entirely satisfactory passage of large stools within hours of the administration of glucagon. Patients who had suffered frequent loose bowel motions, in some cases as often as twelve times a day and sometimes accompanied by the passage of mucus or blood, returned to normal bowel function within an average period of twelve hours. Abdominal distension disappeared when normal bowel action was restored. Palpable masses in the iliac or pelvic colon disappeared more gradually in periods ranging from twelve hours to fourteen days (mean two days).

The only unfavourable reaction attributable to glucagon was nausea and vomiting, which occurred in four of the eight patients who received fairly rapid injection of 1 mg glucagon in 10 ml of diluent. There was no clinically detectable difference between the results of intermittent injection at four-hourly intervals and continuous infusion, other than that the latter was less disturbing for the patient and easier to administer.

Results of conventional treatment

Response to conventional treatment, although ultimately as satisfactory, was slower – principal symptoms persisting for 1.5 to 6 days, a mean of 4 days, as compared to 12 hours with glucagon (Figure 1).

Further experience with the use of glucagon in the treatment of acute diverticulitis

Despite the absence of valid proof of the efficacy of glucagon, due to failure to obtain a satisfactory placebo with which to conduct controlled trials, the evidence reported above was considered sufficient to warrant continued use and in the past seven years a further 68 patients have received intravenous

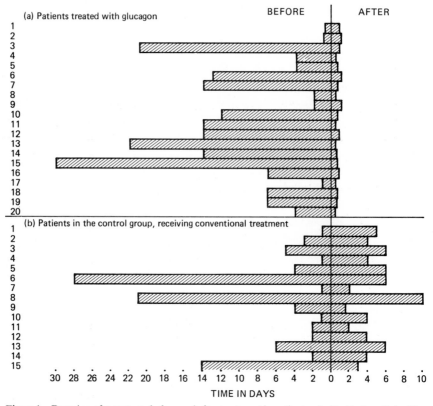

Figure 1 Duration of symptoms before and after treatment in patients admitted to hospital with acute diverticulitis. The upper part of the figure relates to 20 patients treated with intravenous glucagon, the lower section to 15 patients who received conventional treatment for similar symptoms

glucagon as primary treatment of symptoms suggestive of acute diverticulitis. This experience has broadly confirmed the earlier results and provided additional information regarding scope and limitations, as mentioned below.

THE USE OF GLUCAGON TO CONTROL BLEEDING DUE TO DIVERTICULAR DISEASE OF THE COLON

The reported incidence of rectal bleeding in patients admitted to hospital for treatment of diverticular disease of the colon ranges from 11.6 to 21.6 %[13–15], and that of massive bleeding requiring repeated blood transfusion or emergency operation from 3 to 4 %[13]. In the latter group mortality is high[15]. The cause of the bleeding may be ulceration of the artery or vein always present at the neck of diverticulae and separated from the lumen of the bowel by mucous membrane only[16]. Perhaps more frequently, bleeding originates from inflamed mucosa present in the spastic segment of sigmoid colon[13]. Management of severe rectal bleeding associated with diverticular disease often presents a problem because of senility or obesity and if surgery is contemplated by difficulty of identification of the site of bleeding when colonic diverticulae are widespread.

In the eight-year period ending in December 1980, the author's surgical unit admitted a total of eleven patients suffering profuse rectal bleeding due to diverticulitis or diverticular disease. Each required transfusion of two or more units of blood. Four of the eleven were grossly obese, one fifty-year-old man weighing 121 kg. The others were all frail septa- or octogenarians. Each patient received the necessary resuscitative measures and in addition a continuous intravenous infusion of glucagon at a rate of 1 mg every four hours. Rectal bleeding stopped completely within 8 to 18 hours of the commencement of glucagon infusion in all but one patient. In this patient, who presented with a large tender mass in the left iliac fossa, bleeding was much diminished after 12 hours but persisted slightly over the next five days.

THE USE OF GLUCAGON FOR THE RELIEF OF DRUG-INDUCED CONSTIPATION AND INTESTINAL OBSTRUCTION

Several groups of drugs often used for the relief of mental depression, hypertension, pain or muscle spasm have powerful inhibitory side effects on intestinal motility. The resulting prolongation of transit time causes desiccation of colonic content and may lead to massive faecal impaction. If unrelieved, drug-induced constipation is followed by spurious diarrhoea or symptoms and signs of intestinal obstruction, including abdominal distension due to excess of faeces in the colon and also to accumulation of fluid and gas in the small intestine. Vomiting and dehydration ensue.

The agents most often incriminated are the tricyclic antidepressants whose properties include an anticholinergic (atropine-like) action which antagonizes the effect of acetyl choline released at the endings of the vagi and splanchnic nerves and thus inhibits intestinal motility. Anti-spasmodics such as propantheline bromide and poldine methyl sulphate, which are sometimes used in patients with symptoms of irritable bowel, or parkinsonism, have a similar effect. Clonidine hydrochloride as used for the relief of hypertension has a direct inhibiting effect on smooth musle; as a result constipation is a prominent side effect, and there are a few reports of intestinal obstruction occurring[17]. It is well known that opiate analgesics such as codeine, morphine and diphenoxylate have a constipating effect mediated by increase in the tone of intestinal muscle. Abuse of these drugs may cause intestinal obstruction.

Drug-induced constipation is usually relieved by withdrawing the causative agent and administering laxatives and enemas. When the condition is long-standing and obstructive features are present management can be very difficult particularly if enemeta are ineffective. These patients are often mentally disturbed, unable to give a reliable history, and as obstructive symptoms progress laparotomy is sometimes undertaken to exclude other pathology. Such surgery only aggravates the problem and carries a high morbidity and mortality.

The ability of glucagon to relieve colospasm and aid emptying of the bowel offers a new therapeutic possibility especially as glucagon has been shown to inhibit colonic spasm induced by variety of agents, including anti-cholinergic drugs[11,18].

Glucagon has been used successfully on five occasions by the author for the relief of drug-induced constipation or obstruction. As an example, the case is quoted of a 75-year-old woman who was transferred from a mental hospital with symptoms and signs of intestinal obstruction. The patient, who had suffered bouts of constipation for many years, had received 75 mg amitriptyline daily during the previous six weeks as treatment for a severe mental depression. There had been no bowel movement for a week. On the day prior to admission to the surgical unit the abdomen had become distended and vomiting had commenced, first of 'coffee grounds' and later of faecalent fluid. The distended abdomen was tense and tender all over. The rectum was packed with hard scybylae. There were signs of dehydration. X-ray of the abdomen showed distended small bowel with multiple fluid levels and distension of the colon with impacted faeces. Repeated enemas returned faecal stained fluid only. The naso-gastric tube drained up to 2 litres of faecalent fluid daily. In view of the progressive deterioration laparotomy was performed three days after admission to the surgical unit. The whole of the small intestine was dilated with fluid and gas. The colon from caecum to rectum was distended with impacted masses of hard faeces. On the third post-operative day bowel sounds returned but no flatus passed. Infusion of glucagon was then commenced at a rate of 1 mg every four hours and continued for 48 hours. After eight hours passage of flatus occurred and within eighteen hours, aided by another enema, the passage of a large, constipated motion, following which normal bowel function was restored.

THE USE OF GLUCAGON IN CONJUNCTION WITH SUTURED COLONIC ANASTOMOSES

Leakage at the site of colonic anastomosis is a troublesome complication and amongst the possible causes is spasm in the distal bowel. It is known that intra-colonic pressures of up to 300 mmHg may occur in some individuals[19] and the coincidence of such below an anastomosis with waves of peristaltic activity above could create powerful disruptive forces. The risk is probably greatest when there is diverticular disease with associated hypertrophy of colonic muscle. When operations are performed on the sigmoid colon and there is good access to hypertrophied bowel below the anastomosis, a longitudinal myotomy on the anti-mesenteric border provides a simple and effective safeguard against leakage[20]. This technique has been in routine use by the author over the past 15 years. When operating on the transverse colon, however, approach to the lower segment may be difficult without extending the incision as far as the pubis.

The author has given glucagon to five patients undergoing transverse colectomy for carcinoma when there was radiological evidence of diverticular disease in the sigmoid. Continuous infusion at a rate of 1 mg every 4 hours commenced as soon as sounds of bowel activity reappeared after operation and was continued for 48 hours. The results were satisfactory. Easy bowel action followed within 12 hours of the start of infusion and there was no sign of anastomotic leak.

THE USE OF GLUCAGON AS AN AID TO THE FORMATION OF TERMINAL ILEOSTOMY AFTER PAN PROCTO-COLECTOMY

The formation of a satisfactory terminal ileal stoma requires a projecting stump in which the full thickness of the ileum has been everted so that the projection, which should extend 3 or 4 cm in front of the skin of the abdomen, is entirely covered with healthy mucosa. To achieve this 6 to 8 cm of terminal ileum must be drawn out through the abdominal wall and the full thickness of the distal half everted, or pulled inside out, over the remainder. The process of eversion is often made difficult by spasm and the instruments used to hold the inner core whilst the outer is pulled back to skin level may easily damage these friable structures.

The author has found on all occasions when eversion was difficult that the intravenous injection of 1 mg glucagon was followed within 3 to 4 minutes by relaxation of spasm in the terminal ileum and that eversion could then be performed with the minimum of force. In each case the injection of glucagon was also followed, after the same time interval, by a visually obvious increase in blood supply to the severed end.

THE ROLE OF GLUCAGON IN THE DIFFERENTIAL DIAGNOSIS OF ACUTE COLONIC DISEASE

Colonic diverticulae are common in Western countries. Although rare under the age of 40 the incidence rises to probably one in three in persons over the age of 60 years and increases steadily thereafter[16]. In the majority of subjects the diverticulae remain silent but in the author's practice of general surgery in a district general hospital, where there is no special selection of cases, the manifestations of diverticular disease and its complications are responsible for nearly as many admissions as colo-rectal cancer.

The onset of symptoms is usually due to inflammation arising in the apex of a diverticulum and spreading in the form of a dissecting abscess which may burst into the peritoneal cavity or spread longitudinally outside the bowel wall forming an inflammatory mass, or create an internal fistula. Morson[9] has shown that examination of specimens of colon resected for the relief of troublesome symptoms, diagnosed as diverticulitis, often showed no evidence at all of inflammation and that the basic abnormality was a disorder of muscle function resulting in increase in tone of the muscle layers causing shortening of the bowel with consequent muscular thickening of characteristic pattern. To distinguish between the presence and absence of inflammatory changes Morson uses the terms 'diverticulitis' and 'diverticular disease'. The condition in which colonic diverticulae occur without abdominal symptoms is known as diverticulosis.

The fact that colonic diverticula are so common can create diagnostic problems. Diverticulosis may be a coincidental radiological finding in patients with other colonic disease. Furthermore the manifestations of diverticulitis or diverticular disease may closely mimic those of carcinoma of the colon[21], Crohn's disease[22], or ulcerative colitis[16], and often two or more of these major diseases occur simultaneously in the same patient. Although it is always easy to suspect the presence of diverticulitis or diverticular disease, the diagnosis can be established only by a process of exclusion of other pathology and in this, careful investigation and observation of the course of the disease is essential. Barium enema examination is useful in demonstrating diverticulae but neither this nor the traditional clinical criteria can accurately determine whether or not there is associated inflammation, and a co-existing carcinoma[14] or non-specific colitis may well escape radiological detection. Probably the most dangerous combination of dual pathology is diverticular disease or diverticulosis with unrecognized ulcerative colitis. Symptoms will not subside unless both conditions receive adequate simultaneous treatment and segmental resection alone is very likely to be followed by immediate intense exacerbation of the colitis producing severe malaise, profuse, or exsanguinating bloody diarrhoea, or perforation within hours of the operation. Knowledge of the natural history of the disease is an important aid to diagnosis. The initial acute episodes of diverticulitis or diverticular disease are usually transient and following recovery there may be no further symptoms for twenty or more years[23].

Response of attacks of diverticulitis to conventional treatment, though usually satisfactory, is slow. The early days in which improvement is barely perceptible are trying to the patients and a cause of anxiety to their attendants. The main benefit of glucagon therapy is the rapidity with which symptoms are relieved. If symptoms have not disappeared completely within 36 hours, or having gone soon recur, there is a very high probability of the presence of other pathology, most commonly carcinoma, irreversible diverticular stricture, pericolic abscess, ulcerative colitis, or Crohn's disease. Delayed or incomplete recovery, persistence of a palpable mass or early recurrence of symptoms is thus a spur to urgent investigation and this warning comes sooner and more clearly with glucagon than with conventional treatment.

The ability of a potent relaxant of colospasm to relieve symptoms of diverticular disease is comprehensible. The relief afforded to patients with fever, leukocytosis, an acutely tender mass with muscle guarding or rigidity is more surprising, but clearly both glucagon and conventional therapy can abort an impending if not actual peri-colic abscess. It is, however, unlikely that any form of medical treatment will cure an established peri-colic abscess. For example, a 55-year-old man was admitted in 1972 with severe abdominal pain and a tender mass in the left iliac fossa suggestive of acute diverticulitis. Glucagon infusion was followed by complete recovery within 18 hours. In

1977 the symptoms recurred and again responded to glucagon. In 1981 the patient was admitted to hospital with constipation of two weeks' duration and a tender mass in the left iliac fossa. On this occasion there was no response to glucagon. A barium enema showed diverticulitis with a possible malignant stricture. Sigmoid colectomy was performed and the resected specimen showed distended colon above a tight diverticular stricture with a large peri-colic abscess along the mesenteric border, but no sign of malignancy. Resection was followed by uneventful recovery. Surgery is usually required for the relief of peri-colic abscess or persistent obstructive symptoms due to diverticular stricture.

THE USE OF GLUCAGON IN CONJUNCTION WITH END-TO-END STAPLING DEVICE FOR LOW ANTERIOR COLO-RECTAL ANASTOMOSIS

Harford[24] has successfully administered 2 mg glucagon intravenously to relax spasm of a rectal stump which was so severe as to preclude passage of the end-to-end anastomosis stapling device used for low anterior colo-rectal reconstruction.

Moseson et al.[25] reported glucagon to be a useful adjunct to anastomosis with a stapling device. The rapid intravenous injection of 1 mg glucagon was followed within 5 minutes by increase in diameter of the sigmoid colon from 2.0–2.5 cm to as much as 4–6 cm. This facilitated passage of the stapling device and subsequent removal of the hand-anvil component through the end-to-end anastomosis.

THE USE OF GLUCAGON AS AN ADJUNCT TO HYDROSTATIC REDUCTION OR ILEO-COLIC INTUSSUSCEPTION

Hydrostatic reduction by means of radiologically controlled barium enema is now well established as a primary method of treatment of intussusception in children; the reported success rates with barium enema techniques range from 30 to 80%[26,27], or as low as 19% if diagnosis and treatment are delayed[28].

Fisher and Germann[29] reported two cases in which ileo-colic intussusception was reduced with intramuscular injection of 0.5 mg glucagon followed by a barium enema, when the standard therapeutic enema failed. Hoy, Dunbar and Boles[30] reported that 21 of 25 consecutive episodes of ileo-colic intussusception were successfully reduced by the barium enema technique when supplemented by glucagon in a dose of 0.05 mg/kg given either by intramuscular or intravenous injection. No apparent serious complications occurred from the use of this drug and the comfort of the children seemed enhanced due to elimination of some of the cramping pain as well as ease of filling the colon and small intestine. Following the introduction of glucagon therapy the overall success rate of hydrostatic reduction increased for these authors from a previous 61% to 84%.

Haase and Boles[31] evaluated the effect of glucagon on the hydrostatic reduction of experimentally induced intussusception in a prospective double-blind study on 69 puppies. Although there was no statistical difference in overall reduction rate between animals receiving glucagon and those receiving placebo, glucagon did result in significantly easier reduction and an earlier return of normal vascular supply to the retained apex of the intussusception. The results of this experimental work are compatible with the above reported impression that glucagon aids the reduction of intussusception.

DISCUSSION

It is surprising that the possibility of a therapeutic role for glucagon in the management of a variety of colonic disorders, as well as an adjunct to colonic surgery, has not yet been fully explored by adequate randomized double-blind prospective trials.

The results obtained in the treatment of patients with symptoms suggestive of acute diverticulitis are encouraging, but the use of retrospective data for comparison of therapeutic efficacy is not scientifically reliable, and there is a need for a prospective trial to compare the effect of glucagon with conventional and placebo therapy. There is at present no evidence that the results obtained with glucagon differ in any way from those obtained by conventional means, other than in rapidity of response, ease of administration, and the author's and his staff's clinical impressions that the patients appear happier with glucagon than with any other treatment. As attacks of acute diverticulitis are relatively common in areas where colonic diverticulae are endemic there should be no difficulty in quantifying the time factor. The establishment of the role of glucagon as an adjunct to high or low colonic anastomosis, or to the formation of a terminal ileostomy, or in the treatment of severe bleeding due to diverticular disease, or of drug-induced constipation, presents greater difficulties due to the comparative rarity of some of these conditions and the multiplicity of associated variable factors. Nevertheless, the collation of observations from several centres where colonic diseases are commonly found should eventually show whether or not there is a therapeutic role for glucagon. As the administration of glucagon has proved to be relatively free from complications there is no reason why, in the absence of the known specific contraindications, there should be any hesitation in trying the effect of glucagon before accepting failure of hydrostatic reduction of ileo-colic intussusception or embarking on surgery for the relief of severe bleeding due to diverticular disease or the relief of drug-induced constipation. It should also be better to use glucagon to relieve spasm in the terminal ileum before applying force to produce eversions of the ileal stoma, or force to introduce or withdraw a stapling device from the rectum.

Acknowledgement

The author is most grateful to the editor of the *British Medical Journal* for permission to reproduce information previously published, reference no. 10.

References

1. Miller, R. E., Chernish, S. M., Skucas, J., Rosenak, B. E. and Rodda, B. E. (1974). Hypotonic colon examination with glucagon. *Radiology*, **113**, 555
2. Ek, B. (1979). The use of glucagon in colonoscopy. In Picazo, J. (ed.) *Glucagon in Gastroenterology*, pp. 53–58 (Lancaster: MTP Press)
3. Norfleet, R. G. (1978). Premedication for colonoscopy: Randomized double-blind study of glucagon versus placebo. *Gastrointest. Endosc.*, **24**, 164
4. Foster, G. E., Vellacott, K. D., Balfour, T. W. and Hardcastle, J. D. (1981). Outpatient flexible fibreoptic sigmoidoscopy, diagnostic yield and the value of glucagon. *Br. J. Surg.*, **68**, 463
5. Bond, J. H. and Levitt, M. D. (1980). Effect of glucagon on gastrointestinal blood flow in dogs in hypovolemic shock. *Am. J. Physiol.*, **238**, G434
6. Danford, R. O. (1971). The splanchnic vasoconstrictive effect of digoxin and its reversal by glucagon. In Boley, S. J. (ed.) *Vascular Disorders of the Intestine*, pp. 421–428 (New York: Appleton-Century-Crofts)
7. Levinsky, R. A., Lewis, R. M., Bynum, T. E. and Hanley, H. G. (1975). Digoxin induced intestinal vasoconstriction. The effects of proximal arterial stenosis and glucagon administration. *Circulation*, **52**, 130
8. Painter, N. S. (1962). Diverticulosis of the colon. *MS Thesis*, University of London
9. Morson, B. C. (1963). The muscle abnormality in diverticular disease of the sigmoid colon. *Br. J. Radiol.*, **36**, 385
10. Daniel, O., Basu, P. K. and Al-Samarrae, H. (1974). The use of glucagon in the treatment of acute diverticulitis. *Br. Med. J.*, **3**, 720
11. Dotevall, G. and Kock, N. G. (1963). The effect of glucagon on intestinal motility in man. *Gastroenterology*, **45**, 364
12. Necheles, H., Sporn, J. and Walker, L. (1966). Effect of glucagon on gastrointestinal motility. *Am. J. Gastroenterol.*, **45**, 34
13. Bevan, P. G. (1961). Acute diverticulitis: A review of emergency admissions. *Br. Med. J.*, **1**, 400
14. Parks, T. G., Connell, A. M., Gough, A. D. and Cole, J. O. Y. (1970). Limitations of radiology in the differentiation of diverticulitis and diverticulosis of the colon. *Br. Med. J.*, **2**, 136

15. Muir, E. G. (1966). Diverticulitis. *Lancet*, **1**, 195
16. Morson, B. C. (1979). Diverticular disease of the colon. *Acta Chir. Belgica*, **78**, 369
17. George, C. F. (1981). Drugs causing constipation and intestinal obstruction. *Prescribers' Journal*, **21**, 148
18. Chowdhury, A. R. and Lorber, S. H. (1976). The effect of glucagon on cholinomunetic responses of the recto-sigmoid. *GEN (Caracas)*, **31**, 5
19. Daniel, O. (1961). The complications which follow diversion of the urinary stream. *Ann. Roy. Coll. Surg. Eng.*, **29**, 205
20. Reilly, M. C. T. (1979). The place of sigmoid myotomy in diverticular disease. *Acta Chir. Belgica*, **78**, 387
21. Colcock, B. P. and Sass, R. E. (1954). Diverticulitis and carcinoma of the colon: Differential diagnosis. *Surg. Gynecol. Obstet.*, **99**, 627
22. Schmidt, G. T., Lennard-Jones, J. E., Morson, B. C. and Young, A. C. (1968). Crohn's disease of the colon and its distinction from diverticulitis. *Gut*, **9**, 7
23. Bolt, D. E. and Hughes, L. E. (1966). Diverticulitis: A follow-up of 100 cases. *Br. Med. J.*, **1**, 1205
24. Harford, F. J. Jr. (1979). Use of glucagon in conjunction with the end-to-end anastomosis (EEA) stapling device for low anterior anastomoses. *Dis. Colon Rect.*, **22**, 452
25. Moseson, M. D., Hoexter, B. and Labow, S. B. (1980). Glucagon, a useful adjunct in anastomosis with a stapling device. *Dis. Colon Rect.*, **23**, 25
26. Franken, E. A. Jr. (1975). *Gastro-intestinal Radiology in Paediatrics* (Hagerstown, Maryland: Harper & Row)
27. Gierup, J., Jorulf, H. and Livaditis, A. (1972). Management of intussusception in infants and children: A survey based on 288 consecutive cases. *Paediatrics*, **50**, 535
28. Raudkivi, P. J. and Smith, H. L. M. (1981). Intussusception: Analysis of 98 cases. *Br. J. Surg.*, **68**, 645
29. Fisher, J. K. and Germann, D. R. (1977). Glucagon aided reduction of intussusception. *Radiology*, **122**, 197
30. Hoy, G. R., Dunbar, D. and Boles, E. T. Jr. (1977). The use of glucagon in the diagnosis and management of ileocolic intussusception. *J. Paediatr. Surg.*, **12**, 939
31. Haase, G. M. and Boles, E. T. Jr. (1979). Glucagon in experimental intussusception. *J. Paediatr. Surg.*, **14**, 664

Address for correspondence

Dr. O. Daniel,
Ysbyty Glan Clwyd, Bodelwyddan,
Rhyl,
Clwyd LL18 5UJ, UK.

DISCUSSION

Jaspan: Dr. Daniel, may I just recap? What are the doses of glucagon you are using for acute diverticulitis, and is this given as a bolus or as an infusion?

Daniel: We started with a bolus of 1 mg glucagon given fairly quickly, which often resulted in nausea and vomiting. A bolus of 1 mg given slowly over, say, 8 minutes was found to be better tolerated, but we now find that the most satisfactory way of administering the glucagon is by means of a continuous pump which administers it at the rate of 1 mg every four hours.

Jaspan: This is a very high dose.

Christiansen: I was interested in your comments on your use of glucagon when constructing ileostomies. When one is constructing a continent ileostomy reservoir one sometimes has difficulties intubating the reservoir; glucagon is often helpful in such cases. Similarly, it has been reported from the United States that glucagon is helpful when there is a spasm of the intestine when one is performing a stapling anastomosis (Harford, F. J. (1979). *Dis. Colon Rectum*, **22**, 452; Moseson, M. D. *et al.* (1980). *Dis. Colon Rectum*, **23**, 25). And now to the question: Why have you not performed a controlled study on the effect of glucagon in diverticular disease?

Daniel: Simply because we could not obtain a proper placebo at the time. In the absence of a placebo indistinguishable in appearance from the active substance we had to drop the idea of a controlled study. It now seems that it is possible to get a suitable placebo. I agree with you that this is a study which certainly needs to be done, and it could be done very quickly. Such patients are very common nowadays, and I think that in a matter of a year or-so we could probably produce some data.

Miller: Two small comments: firstly, in bleeding we use technetium-99 sulphacolloid to localize the bleeding in order that it can be treated either with drugs that will constrict the blood vessels, or something of that nature. This can be given either by catheter or intravenously. Secondly, it has not yet been mentioned here, but in the United States glucagon is used almost routinely when there is resection of a polyp. This is because one needs the colon to be quiet during the time of resection. If there is spasm and motility of the gut, and the opposite wall of the gut touches the polyp, the current will be transmitted through to the bowel wall, and cause a perforation. Almost all our endoscopists doing colonoscopic polyp resection now use glucagon to quiet the bowel wall.

Skucas: During colonoscopy, especially when the colonoscopist is passing through the sigmoid and performing the alpha manoeuvre the sigmoid becomes stretched and some people believe that it is the stretching of the sigmoid mesentery which actually results in pain to the patient. Glucagon probably does not have any effect upon this particular type of pain. Secondly, some colonoscopists like a little tonicity in the colon, so that the colon more or less intussuscepts on the colonoscope. They feel that this helps them to reach the caecum a little faster.

Vilardell: Several years ago I was quite impressed by some observations published in a British journal concerning what happened to the colon when neostigmine was given to reverse the effects of muscle relaxants after colonic surgery (Bell, C. M. A. and Lewis, C. B. (1968). *Br. Med. J.*, **3**, 587). Striking spasm of the colon could be demonstrated in some cases, and the incidence of anastomotic leaks was much greater in patients having neostigmine than in a control group of subjects who did not have the drug. The effect of neostigmine was later confirmed by manometric studies (Wilkins, J. L. *et al.* (1970). *Br. Med. J.*, **3**, 793). I wonder if glucagon might be useful in this spastic situation and whether it could be of any help in preventing anastomotic leakage. My second point is that you reported on two series of patients, Dr. Daniel, one was the current series where you gave glucagon, and the other was a previous series of patients seen retrospectively. You compared a lot of data, and saw quite an impressive difference in a number of symptoms. There may be differences in small things that do not really mean much, but other things are very important. What are the symptoms you would pay more attention to, if you had to choose just two or three, in order to decide that your patients do better when given glucagon. Would pain be one?

Daniel: The striking thing is that with glucagon the patients appear 'much happier'. It is a little difficult to define. You see, with the conventional treatment the patients remain in pain and discomfort for many days whilst receiving treatment. The pain can be partly suppressed, maybe by pethidine, but glucagon seems not so much to suppress the symptoms as to relieve the actual cause. So that, and the speed with which pain and discomfort disappear, I think are the two main things.

Vilardell: A final question. One of the side effects of glucagon one occasionally sees is vomiting. This would not be a particularly desirable thing in a patient in acute abdominal pain due to diverticulitis.

Daniel: Vomiting would indeed complicate matters, but one now avoids that by giving the glucagon more slowly. When this is done there seem to be no side effects at all.

7

The use of endoscopic manometry to demonstrate the effect of glucagon on the sphincter of Oddi

J.-F. REY, J. CORALLO, J. LOMBART and J. PANGTAY-TEA

The sphincter of Oddi has been the subject of much study[1,2] since it was first described by Ruggiero Oddi in 1887[3]. In spite of numerous animal studies, however, the physiology and pathology of the human sphincter of Oddi have remained rather poorly understood. Among the facts which are known are the various effects of cholecystokinin[4-6], of prostaglandins[7], of adrenergic hormones[8], and of gastrointestinal polypeptides[9,10], all of which are known to affect the delivery of bile to the duodenum[11].

Until relatively recently investigators wishing to study the sphincter of Oddi had to do so during surgery or by means of T-tube radiomanometry[12,13] or cine-radiography[14]. Since the mid-1970s, however, particularly since the development of a side-viewing duodenoscope[15], it has been possible to study this sphincter during endoscopic retrograde cholangiopancreatography (ERCP). Several teams of investigators have published their findings (Table 1)[16-22].

This method of investigation, endoscopic manometry, is however still in its infancy; even now, despite important improvements in the course of the last five or so years, it is by no means problem-free. Carr-Locke and Gregg have

Table 1 Pressures recorded in control subjects by means of endoscopic manometry. The data are expressed in mmHg. The table shows the basal pressures recorded in the sphincter of Oddi (SO), the common bile duct (CBD), and the pancreatic duct (PD), and the pressure gradients between the common bile duct and the duodenum (D), the pancreatic duct and the duodenum, and the common bile duct and the sphincter of Oddi. The figures in brackets indicate the peak pressures reached during phasic contractions of the sphincter of Oddi

Report	SO	CBD	PD	CBD/D	PD/D	CBD/SO
Nebel, 1975[16]	31	—	—	—	—	—
Rösch et al., 1976[17]	—	23.8	22.2	—	—	—
Hagenmüller et al., 1977[18]	31	19.7	—	—	—	—
Geenen et al., 1977[19]	—	—	—	9.3	4	4
Bar-Meir et al., 1979[20]	49 (149)	27	30	12	15	22
Geenen et al., 1980[21]	31 (101)	27.4	30.4	12.4	15.7	4
Carr-Locke and Gregg, 1981[22]	31 (62.6)	18	31	3	16	13
Rey et al., 1982	35.5	28.2	32.5	15.3	19.6	7.3

recently drawn attention to some of the difficulties involved.[22] One of the factors which has a direct effect on the pressures recorded is the infusion rate used. Marked differences have been found in the range tested, 0.12 ml/min to 1.23 ml/min. A rate of 0.23 ml/min, for example, has been found to result in the recording of pressure peaks only 53 % as high as those recorded when a rate of 0.62 ml/min is used. It is likely that the use of different infusion rates accounts for at least some of the differences in the pressures reported to date by different teams of investigators (Table 1).

Geenen et al.[21] have similarly attributed the recording of different results to the use of differing systems of instrumentation. In 1979 these authors were the first, using endoscopic manometry, to record phasic contractions in the human sphincter of Oddi[20,21]. They did so when using a new developed minimally compliant hydraulic-capillary system to infuse the catheters[23]. In all previous studies this had been done by means of a high compliant syringe pump. Geenen and his co-workers concluded that with the conventionally used infusion system the phasic contractions had either been inapparent or so dampened that their importance had not been recognized.

The use of a minimally compliant infusion system does indeed lead to the production of more detailed, and therefore more accurate, recordings. There is a problem, however, in that when such a system is used there is a considerable increase in the amount of background interference, and the tracings can therefore be difficult to interpret. Artifacts are still a tremendous problem in investigations of this sort, and in practice it is wise to make several recordings in each case in order to minimize the effect of these.

Despite the complexities, endoscopic manometry has added greatly to our knowledge of the physiology of the human sphincter of Oddi. It has also provided a means of accurately recording the actions of hormones on this sphincter.

The spasmolytic effect of glucagon, already apparent from other types of study, has been confirmed and quantitated by endoscopic manometry (Table 2)[21,24,25]. It is effective in doses as low as 0.2 mg i.v.[21]. Cholecystokinin, 0.02 µg/kg i.v., has been found to markedly reduce or even abolish sphincter of Oddi activity[5,21]. It works speedily, its spasmolytic effect becoming evident within 30 seconds. This effect has not been found very useful in clinical practice, however, as at the same time as relaxing the sphincter of Oddi, cholecystokinin contracts the gallbladder and dramatically increases duodenal motility. It also induces unpleasant side effects, such as nausea and vomiting. Secretin, 1 U/kg i.v., has been found to have a biphasic effect on the sphincter of Oddi: first, after 3 min, there is an increase in pressure, and then, after 6 min, a decrease to below control levels[21]. Both cholecystokinin and secretin stimulate biliary and pancreatic secretion; their use therefore increases fluid flow across the sphincter.

Most of the hormonal studies reported to date have been conducted in healthy control subjects. Evidence of the effects of these hormones, however, leads one to wonder if they might not be of therapeutic value in some cases of sphincter of Oddi abnormalities. It was for this reason that when planning our own study – which is basically in healthy subjects, for the amount of published

Table 2 Effect of glucagon on sphincter of Oddi pressure in control subjects

Report	No. of patients	Dose	Sphincter of Oddi pressure after administration of glucagon
Geenen et al., 1980[21]	8	0.4 mg	Reduced by 3–5 mmHg
	4	0.2 mg	Reduced by 20–30%
Classen, 1981[24]	6	0.5 mg	Reduced
Viceconte, 1981[25]	5	0.5 mg	2 Reduced by 30%
			3 No change
Rey et al., 1982	15	1 mg	Reduced by 30–50% (mean value 34%)

data is still somewhat small – we decided to include some patients with sphincter of Oddi disorders. Our own interest and experience, as well as that of others[17, 26], led to the decision to include two types of patient: (a) those diagnosed as suffering stenosis of the sphincter of Oddi, in whom no stones were apparent, and (b) those who had undergone endoscopic sphincterotomy. In view of previously published findings, we decided to study the effect of glucagon on this occasion. The somewhat high dose of 1 mg i.v. was chosen in order to ensure maximum effect. Our study is at an early stage, but we should like to report the data obtained so far.

METHOD

The method being used is basically that described by Geenen et al.[21]. It is illustrated in Figure 1. All subjects are lightly sedated for the ERCP examination with diazepam, 10 mg i.v., which has been shown to have no effect on the sphincter of Oddi[27]. The duodenoscope used is the newly designed Olympus JF-1T. Two types of catheter are used: a standard Olympus catheter with two side holes, and a catheter with a sealed tip and one side hole, which Carr-Locke and Gregg[22] have found to greatly facilitate the accurate recording of pressures in the sphincter of Oddi. These are catheters B and C in Figure 2. A low compliance hydraulic-capillary pump is used to infuse the catheters with a sterile 0.9 % saline solution. The infusion rate is 0.5 ml/min. The pressures are transmitted to a Thomson transducer and transcribed on a Sarinco recorder.

Pressure recordings are made in three positions: (a) in the common bile duct with the catheter inserted deep in the bile duct, (b) in the sphincter of Oddi with

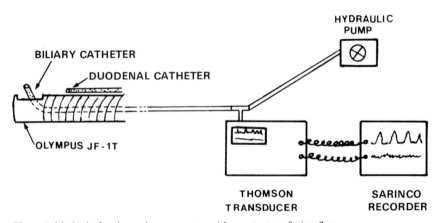

Figure 1 Method of endoscopic manometry with constant perfusion flow

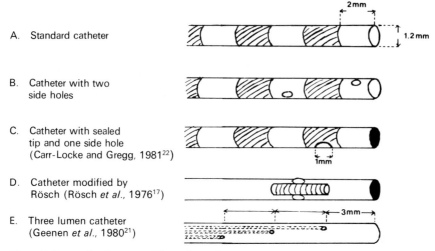

Figure 2 Types of catheters used for endoscopic manometry

the catheter positioned between the two main sections[2], and (c) in the duodenum. Each measurement is made three times in each subject in an attempt to avoid misinterpretation of the situation due to artifacts.

The correct positioning of the catheters is checked by endoscopic control, and, in the case of the measurement in the common bile duct, by the drawing of yellow bile. During the first ten examinations a second catheter was attached to the exterior of the duodenoscope in order to make a continuous recording of the pressure in the duodenum. This practice was abandoned when it was found that the pressure in the duodenum remained constant throughout, and could therefore be recorded by the manometric catheter.

In most cases the pressures have been recorded before and after the administration of glucagon, 1 mg i.v. The glucagon is administered via an intravenous catheter which is kept in place throughout the endoscopic procedure. It is injected slowly in order to avoid the nausea and vomiting which might otherwise occur. To date, no side effects have been seen as the result of the use of glucagon, nor have any subjects or patients reacted adversely to the ERCP examination.

RESULTS

(a) Control subjects

In 14 subjects we first recorded just the basal common bile duct and duodenum pressures. We found average pressures of 28.2 mmHg in the common bile duct

103

and of 12.9 mmHg in the duodenum, a gradient therefore of 15.3 mmHg (Figure 3).

Using the above-described method we then measured the phasic contractions of the sphincter of Oddi. In Figure 4 we reproduce a manometric recording made in a control subject as the recording catheter was drawn from the common bile duct, through the sphincter of Oddi, and into the duodenum. This clearly shows a steady basal pressure, of 34.5 mmHg, in the common bile duct, phasic contractions in the sphincter of Oddi with major peaks rising to 108 mmHg and occurring at the rate of 3 per minute, and a steady pressure, of 12.7 mmHg, in the duodenum. The lower tracing in this figure was recorded by a catheter attached to the duodenoscope; it shows that the pressure in the duodenum remained steady throughout the investigation.

In 15 subjects we then recorded the pressures in the common bile duct, the sphincter of Oddi, and the duodenum, both before and after the administration of glucagon (1 mg i.v.). In these subjects we found that glucagon lowered the sphincter of Oddi pressure by 34%, from an average of 38.2 mmHg to one of 25.4 mmHg (Table 3). It reduced the common bile duct pressure by 47%, from an average of 29.1 mmHg to one of 15.3 mmHg (Table 3). The effect in both areas began 2 minutes after administration and lasted for

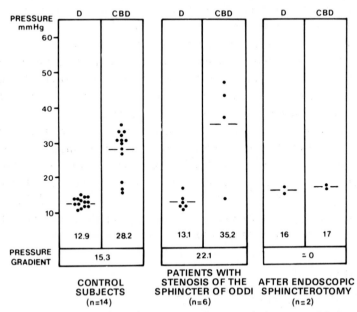

Figure 3 Basal recordings by endoscopic manometry of pressures in the common bile duct (CBD) and the duodenum (D) in control subjects, in patients with stenosis of the sphincter of Oddi, and in patients having undergone endoscopic sphincterotomy

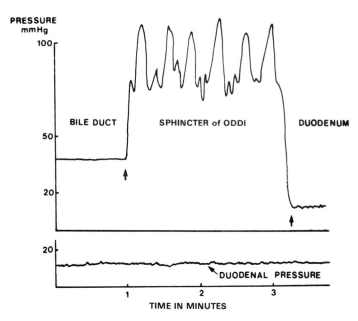

Figure 4 Manometric recording of station pull-through from the common bile duct, through the sphincter of Oddi, to the duodenum. The upper tracing shows the pressure recorded by a pull-through catheter; the arrows indicate the common bile duct/sphincter of Oddi junction and the sphincter of Oddi/duodenum junction. The lower tracing, recorded at the same time, came from a catheter attached to the exterior of the duodenoscope

8–10 minutes. The sphincter of Oddi waves were almost completely abolished for 3–4 minutes. The administration of glucagon also led to the relaxation of the duodenum; an effect which began 90 seconds after administration.

(b) Patients with stenosis of the sphincter of Oddi

It is difficult to perform endoscopic manometry in patients suffering stenosis of the sphincter of Oddi. Deep cannulation is often impossible in such cases unless anti-spasmodic agents are used. In 3 of the cases in which we have so far succeeded in measuring both the common bile duct pressure and the duodenal pressure we have found the common bile duct pressure to be remarkably high (Figure 3). Carr-Locke and Gregg[22] have reported a similar finding. To date we have measured the common bile duct pressure and the sphincter of Oddi pressure before and after the administration of glucagon in five cases. In 3

105

Table 3 Pressures in the sphincter of Oddi (SO) and in the common bile duct (CBD) before and after the administration of glucagon, 1 mg i.v. The data are expressed in mmHg

	SO		CBD	
	Before glucagon	After glucagon	Before glucagon	After glucagon
Control subjects	38.2	25.4	29.1	15.3
($n = 15$)				
Patients with stenosis of the sphincter of Oddi	54.9	41.9	32.1	28.5
($n = 5$)		($n = 3$)		($n = 3$)
		52.1		33.4
		($n = 2$)		($n = 2$)
After endoscopic sphincterotomy, and after the administration of morphine, 10 mg s.c.	16.4	13.1	14.1	13.8
($n = 7$)				

glucagon resulted in a moderate decrease in the sphincter of Oddi pressure, but in the other 2 an effect was barely discernible (Table 3); in no instances has a real spasmolytic effect been seen. Similar results have been reported by Bar-Meir et al.[20] and by Viceconte[25]. These findings reflect our ERCP experience: in cases in which biliary cannulation is difficult we have found glucagon to be helpful in some 80% of cases in which the problem is due to spasmodic contraction of the sphincter of Oddi, but of no help when the problem is due to fibrous stenosis.

(c) Post-sphincterotomy

We have so far used endoscopic manometry to check the post-sphincterotomy situation in seven patients. In each case the sphincter of Oddi had been completely cut. The result, of course, is that the common bile duct pressure is markedly impaired and the common bile duct to duodenum pressure gradient practically non-existent (Figure 3). The administration of morphine in such cases leads to a constriction of the remnant biliary infundibulum and, therefore, to an increase both in the common bile duct pressure and in the common bile duct to duodenum pressure gradient[28]. Accordingly we administered morphine, 10 mg s.c., to five patients and then measured the pressures in the biliary infundibulum, the sphincter superior[2], and the duodenum. We found that the subsequent administration of glucagon, 1 mg i.v., to these patients resulted in a reduction of the morphine-induced pressure increases in the common bile duct and in the sphincter of Oddi (Table 3), and therefore in a reduction in the morphine-induced common bile duct to duodenum pressure gradient.

COMMENTS

It is clear that in endoscopic manometry we have an extremely useful means of measuring pressures in the sphincter of Oddi and in neighbouring organs. Its use has provided confirmation of the descriptions of the sphincter of Oddi given to us by surgeons and pathologists, and added considerably to our knowledge of the motor activity of this sphincter. Its use has also enabled accurate recordings to be made of the effects of several hormones; its particular value here lies in the fact that it allows one to measure the activity within the sphincter itself, unhampered by changes in bile flow or in duodenal activity.

Recent developments, namely the introduction of a low compliant hydraulic-capillary infusion system and modifications to the design of the catheters, have greatly improved the detail and accuracy of the recordings obtained by endoscopic manometry, but care must be taken with the interpretation of the resultant data, as, at least at present, artifacts appear almost inherent in recordings of this type. The fact that different results are obtained by even slightly differing techniques also makes it difficult to compare the data of one centre with those of another; it is important that each patient be compared with control group data recorded by precisely the same method[29]. It is estimated, incidentally, that even if one was able to eliminate all known interfering factors, artifacts would still appear in some 5–10% of recordings.

As far as glucagon is concerned, endoscopic manometry has confirmed and quantitated its spasmolytic action on the sphincter of Oddi and on the duodenum. The effect is dose-related, but appears to be maximal at a dose level of 1 mg i.v. In clinical practice we have tried a second injection some 10 minutes later when the first has been ineffective, but without success. Results similar to those obtained by us in control subjects have been reported by Classen[24], Geenen et al.[21], and Viceconte[25] (Table 2).

It is clearly too early to talk about any therapeutic effects which the continuous administration of glucagon might have in cases of sphincter of Oddi disorders. Paul[30], however, has reported glucagon to be useful in stimulating the passage of stones after endoscopic sphincterotomy, and also in

107

cases of residual microlithiasis when the papilla has been intact. It has been found useful for relaxing the duodenum during ERCP, and for relaxing the sphincter of Oddi during cannulation. In the United States it is routinely used during endoscopic practice.

It would be interesting to know the value of the combination of endoscopic manometry and glucagon in cases of juxtapapillary diverticuli; Osnes et al.[31] have found an increase in choledocholithiasis in such cases, and Funch-Jenssen et al.[32] have found bacterial overgrowth.

Could endoscopic manometry resolve the discussion between clinicians about spasm of the sphincter of Oddi versus odditis? It is doubtful, as many patients with suspected odditis have functional disorders, not organic ones. If true benign stenosis does exist it probably represents less than 10% of the cases referred to a highly specialized department. Nevertheless, just as one has to treat 'irritable bowel disease', so one has to try to relieve 'irritable biliary syndrome', by using drugs not surgery.

It is likely that the next major step forward will be made by using the techniques of endoscopic manometry for electromyographic studies. Ono[33] and Bourgeon et al.[34] have already shown the sphincter of Oddi to have an electrical activity, one which appears to be independent of that of the duodenum. Work in this field is held up at the moment by technical problems, it being difficult to insert the electrodes without damaging either them or the duodenoscope. Hopes are high, however, that this problem will soon be resolved.

In conclusion, it may be said that in endoscopic manometry we now have an extremely useful means of studying the human sphincter of Oddi. Endoscopic manometric studies have added greatly to our knowledge of the motor activity of this sphincter, and of the effect of several hormones on this activity. This method of investigation would clearly enable a speedy and accurate assessment to be made of any therapies designed to alleviate problems caused by sphincter of Oddi disorders. If such a therapy is to involve the use of any of the hormones tested to date, it would seem that glucagon, with its synergistic relaxing action on the sphincter of Oddi and on the duodenum, would be a strong candidate.

Acknowledgement

The authors acknowledge with respect the work of Professor L. Barraya in connection with the sphincter of Oddi, and wish to record their appreciation to him for his help in their early days of endoscopic practice.

References

1. Boyden, E. A. (1965). The comparative anatomy of the sphincter of Oddi in mammals, with special reference to the choledochoduodenal junction in man. In Taylor, W. (ed.) *The Biliary System. A Symposium of the NATO Advanced Study Institute*, pp. 15–40 (Oxford: Blackwell)
2. Barraya, L., Pujol-Soler, R. and Yvergneaux, J. P. (1971). La région Oddienne anatomie millimétrique. *Presse Méd.*, **79**, 2527
3. Oddi, R. (1887). D'une disposition à sphincter spéciale de l'ouverture du canal cholédoque. *Arch. Ital. Biol.*, **8**, 317
4. Lin, T. M. and Spray, G. F. (1969). Effect of pentagastrin, cholecystokinin, caerulein and glucagon on the choledochal resistance and bile flow in dogs. *Gastroenterology*, **56**, 1178 (Abstract)
5. Rey, J.-F. and Harvey, R. F. (1977). Hormonal control of the sphincter of Oddi. In Delmont, J. (ed.) *The Sphincter of Oddi*, pp. 66–71 (Basel: Karger)
6. Behar, J. and Biancani, P. (1980). Effect of cholecystokinin and the octapeptide of cholecystokinin on the feline sphincter of Oddi and gallbladder. *J. Clin. Invest.*, **66**, 1231
7. Nakata, K. and Kurahashi (1981). Effects of C terminal octapeptide of cholecystokinin and prostaglandins on adrenergic functions in the guinea-pig gallbladder and sphincter of Oddi. *Jpn. J. Pharmacol.*, **31**, 77
8. Persson, C. G. A. (1972). Adrenergic, cholecystokinetic and morphine-induced effects on extra-hepatic motility. *Acta Physiol. Scand.* (suppl.) **383**, 4
9. Lin, T. M. (1975). Action of gastrointestinal hormones and related peptides on the motor function of the biliary tract. *Gastroenterology*, **69**, 1006
10. Toouli, J. and Watts, J. M. (1972). Actions of cholecystokinin/pancreozymin, secretin and gastrin on extra-hepatic biliary tract motility in vitro. *Ann. Surg.*, **175**, 439
11. Askrim, J. R., Lyon, D. T., Shull, S. D., Wagner, C. I. and Soloway, R. D. (1978). Factors affecting delivery of bile to the duodenum in man. *Gastroenterology*, **74**, 560
12. Bonfils, S., Gislon, J. and Galmiche, J. P. (1974). Manométrie biliaire post-opératoire sous perfusion intracholédocienne à débuts variés avec ou sans administration de morphine. *Biol. Gastroentérol.*, **7**, 117
13. Treffot, M.-J., Quilichini, F. and Vinson, M.-F. (1979). Biliary surgery, radiomanometry and glucagon. In Picazo, J. (ed.) *Glucagon in Gastroenterology*, pp. 87–93 (Lancaster: MTP Press)
14. Caroli, J., Porcher, G., Pequignot, G. and Delattre, M. (1960). Contribution of cine-radiography to study of the function of the human biliary tract. *Am. J. Dig. Dis.*, **5**, 677
15. Cotton, P. B. (1977). E.R.C.P. *Gut*, **18**, 316
16. Nebel, O. T. (1975). Effect of enteric hormones on the human sphincter of Oddi. *Gastroenterology*, **68**, 105 (Abstract)
17. Rösch, W., Koch, H. and Demling, L. (1976). Manometric studies during E.R.C.P. and endoscopic papillotomy. *Endoscopy*, **8**, 30
18. Hagenmüller, P., Ossenberg, F. W. and Classen, M. (1977). Duodenoscopic manometry of the common bile duct. In Delmont, J. (ed) *The Sphincter of Oddi*, pp. 72–76 (Basel: Karger)
19. Geenen, J. E., Hogan, W. J., Shaffer, R. D., Stewart, E. T., Dodds, W. J. and Arndorfer, R. C. (1977). Endoscopic electrosurgical papillotomy and manometry in biliary tract disease. *J. Am. Med. Assoc.*, **237**, 2075
20. Bar-Meir, S., Geenen, J. E., Hogan, W. J., Dodds, W. J., Stewart, E. T. and Arndorfer, R. C. (1979). Biliary and pancreatic duct pressures measured by E.R.C.P. manometry in patients with suspected papillary stenosis. *Dig. Dis. Sci.*, **24**, 209
21. Geenen, J. E., Hogan, W. J., Dodds, W. J., Stewart, E. T. and Arndorfer, R. C. (1980). Intraluminal pressure recording from the human sphincter of Oddi. *Gastroenterology*, **78**, 317
22. Carr-Locke, D. L. and Gregg, J. A. (1981). Endoscopic manometry of pancreatic and biliary sphincter zones in man. Basal results in healthy volunteers. *Dig. Dis. Sci.*, **26**, 7
23. Arndorfer, R. C., Stef, J. J., Dodds, W. J., Linehan, J. H. and Hogan, W. J. (1977). Improved

infusion system for intraluminal esophageal manometry. *Gastroenterology*, **73**, 23

24. Classen, M. (1981). Endoscopic approach to papillary stenosis. *Endoscopy*, **13**, 154
25. Viceconte, G. (1981). Endoscopic manometry of the sphincter of Oddi. Presented at the IIIème Symposium International d'Endoscopie Digestive, May 30, Paris
26. Ribeiro, B. F., Cotton, P. B., Dilawari, J. B., Roberts, M. and Laurence, B. (1977). Duodenoscopic manometry of the bile duct and sphincter of Oddi. *Gut*, **18**, A406 (Abstract)
27. Nebel, O. T. (1975). Manometric evaluation of the papilla of Vater. *Gastrointest. Endosc.*, **21**, 126
28. Rey, J.-F., Pangtay-Tea, J. and Ljunggren, B. (1977). Endoscopic control of surgical sphincteroplasty of the sphincter of Oddi. In Delmont, J. (ed.) *The Sphincter of Oddi*, pp. 213–218 (Basel: Karger)
29. Tanaka, M., Ikeda, S. and Nakayama, F. (1981). Non-operative measurement of pancreatic and common bile duct pressures with a microtransducer catheter and effects of duodenoscopic sphincterotomy. *Dig. Dis. Sci.*, **26**, 545
30. Paul, F. (1979). The role of glucagon in the treatment of biliary tract pathology. In Picazo, J. (ed.) *Glucagon in Gastroenterology*, pp. 107–118. (Lancaster: MTP Press)
31. Osnes, M., Myren, J., Lotveit, T. and Swensen, T. (1977). Juxtapapillary duodenal diverticula and abnormalities by endoscopic retrograde cholangio-pancreatography. *Scand. J. Gastroenterol.*, **12**, 347
32. Funch-Jenssen, P., Csendes, A., Kruse, A. and Oster, M. J. (1979). Common bile duct pressure and Oddi sphincter pressure in patients with common bile duct stones with and without juxta ampullar diverticula of duodenum. *Scand. J. Gastroenterol.*, **14**, 253
33. Ono, K. (1970). The discharge of bile into the duodenum and electrical activities of the muscle of Oddi and duodenum. *Jpn. J. Smooth Muscle Res.*, **6**, 123
34. Bourgeon, R., Isman, H., Lupo, B., Brisard, M. and Bottau, A. (1979). La synergie duodéno-oddienne chez l'homme. *Méd. Chir. Dig.*, **8**, 629

Address for correspondence:

Dr. J.-F. Rey,
Départment d'Hépatologie et de Gastro-entérologie,
Institut Arnault Tzanck,
Plateaudes Galinières,
06700 Saint Laurent du Var (Nice), France

DISCUSSION

Daniel: Dr Rey's work is a most encouraging indication of the possibility of recognizing and treating an important group of patients without recourse to laparotomy. I refer to those in whom symptoms of upper abdominal pain and often fever and jaundice are strongly suggestive of stone in the common duct, but who on operation are found to have non-calculous disease of which the main pathologic feature is inflammation and stenosis of the papilla of Vater and sphincter of Oddi. The very existence of such pathology is strongly denied by some and apparently unknown to many surgeons, yet in my experience it is found in some 2 % of the mass of patients undergoing operation for suspected gallstones. It seems quite possible that manometric studies performed by endoscopic approach will lead to recognition of this condition and that symptoms may then be relieved by endoscopic papillotomy or sphincterotomy.

Dr Rey drew attention to the difficulties encountered in measuring pressure and these have, no doubt, been responsible for the disappointing results of many investigators. My own approach has been to rely mainly on measurement of rate of flow at low hydrostatic pressure through a relatively wide bored tube (no. 10 Portex Infant Feeding Catheter) introduced into the cystic duct during the course of cholecystectomy, or occasionally directly into the common duct. Changes in the intermittent contraction and relaxation of the sphincter are reflected in the flow rate and the rigidity of the tube is such as to minimize the risks of false results due to kinking. The biliary tract is exquisitely sensitive to physical or pharmacological stimulation. The infusion fluid must be physiological saline at body temperature and all exogenous stimuli minimized for a few minutes prior to and during recording. Misleading results due to iatrogenic spasm may be overcome by the use of glucagon but are best avoided by careful attention to detail. The use of small bore soft walled tubes limits the scope of studies and also increases the risk of false results. The normal bile duct and sphincter can cope with flow rates in excess of 120 ml/min at effective hydrostatic pressure head of 30 cm water. Rates of this magnitude can be achieved only through the use of tubes of 3 mm internal diameter. With these precautions, very valuable observations can be made on the functional state of the complex sphincter mechanism of the biliary tract using very simple apparatus (Daniel, O. (1972). *Ann. R. Coll. Surg. Eng.*, **51**, 357).

Baker: I think this study of Dr. Rey's is a very interesting one and I have a couple of questions from the point of view of a clinician who does not do this kind of work. I wonder if you would say a little more about the variation in the observations that you made from time to time. You alluded to the fact that you found variations in pressures as well as spurious numbers, and I wonder if you could tell us the range of the variability. Also, you showed in one of your figures a ratio between common duct pressure and duodenal pressure which varied quite widely between studies among people using this technique. It would seem that a systematic error would leave you all with the same ratio. I wonder if you could comment a little further about these two points.

Rey: About your second point, I think one must be a little careful when comparing the results of different authors. There have been two major publications, one by Geenen, J. E. *et al.* (1980, *Gastroenterology*, **78**, 317) and one by Carr-Locke, D. L. and Gregg, J. A. (1981, *Dig. Dis. Sci.*, **26**, 7). Both groups use a similar kind of pressure, but with different absolute results. Carr-Locke and Gregg got a 50 mmHg increase and Geenen *et al.* 120 mmHg, but what was important is that they had exactly the same kind of ratio, and that is of significance if you are studying a patient with increase of common bile duct pressure. In my study I did not use the absolute number from either of these studies. I wanted to use my own control. Finally, regarding your question about the variation, the standard error is about 20% in our study. It is quite important.

Baker: How does your system differ from that of others doing similar studies? You use a high fidelity recording channel and a single channel recording catheter. Are these the principal differences?

Rey: The principal difference is in my use of a single channel recording catheter with one side-holed end.

Skucas: What are your indications for endoscopic sphincterotomy?

Rey: My indications for endoscopic sphincterotomy are stones, on many occasions periampullary carcinoma. Benign Oddi stenosis is not a good indication. This is why I set up this kind of system, because, in my opinion, one should be conservative about endoscopic sphincterotomy. Safrany, in his first three hundred endoscopic sphincterotomies, did 30% of them just for benign stenosis (Safrany, L. (1977). *Gastroentrology*, **72**, 338), but we only cut the sphincter when we are sure that there are stones in the common bile duct, or some definite pathology as indicated by a dilated common bile duct, a clinical history of biliary pain, and an elevated common bile duct pressure; but common bile duct pressure is just one of the components along with the clinical and the radiology evidence. I avoid doing sphincterotomy for benign stenosis, and in actual fact in a little over 300 endoscopic sphincterotomies I have only done it on four occasions for that indication.

Skucas: Do you have any follow up data after sphincterotomy?

Rey: Yes, five years' follow up and we have 1.5% of restenosis after endoscopic sphincterotomy.

Jaspan: I would like to make a plea for the use of infusion in all these studies rather than injection. The prime reason for this is the physiology of clearance of glucagon. The half-life is about 4 minutes and I think the therapeutic index can be improved markedly minimizing nausea, vomiting and other side effects. If one needs just a single pharmacologic dose to relax bowel, a bolus injection may, at first, seem more appropriate, but if it results in nausea and vomiting its value will be somewhat limited. One would do much better, I think, to give an injection of 0.1 mg glucagon as Dr. Miller does, followed by an infusion. When a more prolonged period of therapeutic usefulness is envisioned, such as when one is attempting to decrease pressure over a period of time as in diverticular disease, for example, or possibly when trying to dislodge gallstones, I think much more mileage could be got and a much greater therapeutic index by using an infusion at 25 ng/kg per minute or approximately 100 µg/h (0.1 mg/h), which is a pharmacological dose producing glucagon levels some 50 times physiologic (≈ 5 ng/ml) but short of the astronomically high and short lived elevations that will occur with 1 mg bolus injections.

Hardcastle: You clearly demonstrated that there is a group of patients with stenosis of the lower end of the common bile duct. Have you shown that there are patients with spasm producing symptoms? I can understand stenosis which is symptomatic, but do you think spasm of the sphincter of Oddi actually exists?

Rey: I think so, yes. A few patients with spasm of the sphincter of Oddi have biliary pain but I would not perform endoscopic sphincterotomy or surgical sphincterotomy in them.

Hardcastle: How do you treat these patients?

Rey: This is a problem. I try to relax them with drugs. I have found hymecromone quite useful for this purpose.

Vilardell: Biliary tract surgery has a very long history in France, specially since the early fifties, due to the work of Caroli and his group who did manometry through the cystic duct in thousands of patients and sphincterotomies in many of them (Caroli, J. (1956). *Les ictères par rétention.* Paris: Masson). We have done long-term follow ups in many of our operated patients and those who had had sphincterotomies for what seemed to be true disease of the sphincter of Oddi, where all pathologists could see fibrosis and inflammation, did not fare very well with sphincterotomy. I would say, in my own experience, half of them did not do very well at all. They continued to have symptoms.

Rey: Yes, I agree with Prof. Vilardell. I do not think endoscopic or surgical sphincterotomy is justified in cases of benign stenosis or fibrostenosis.

8

The use of glucagon in spastic disorders of the gastrointestinal tract

**J. D. HARDCASTLE, M. J. STOWER and
G. E. FOSTER**

INTRODUCTION

Pancreatic glucagon is a 29 amino acid peptide with a molecular weight of 3485, secreted by the A cells of the pancreas[1]. Under physiological conditions its role is to mobilize hepatic glucose and to stimulate the breakdown of fatty acids and ketone bodies during carbohydrate or total starvation, impending hypoglycaemia or whenever the metabolic demand exceeds exogenous supply[2]. It is not clear whether the effects of glucagon on gastrointestinal function are physiological or only seen when pharmacological doses of the hormone are given.

THE ACTION OF GLUCAGON ON THE BILIARY TRACT

Acute pain originating from the biliary tract arises when a calculus becomes impacted in Hartmann's pouch or cystic duct and painful contractions of the biliary smooth muscle result[3]. Initially this gives rise to acute biliary colic, the gall bladder becoming engorged, tense and undergoing spasmodic contractile activity in an attempt to expel the gall stone. Biliary colic is often initially wrongly labelled as acute cholecystitis when in fact infection is not likely to be present at first, secondary infection supervening only if flow from the gall bladder continues to be obstructed.

Glucagon relaxes the gall bladder of the conscious dog when given either by subcutaneous or intravenous injection, a response which is dose related[4]. Chernish et al.[5] demonstrated that in man glucagon significantly increased the size of the gall bladder when given alone or given after a fatty meal, but this effect could not be demonstrated in vitro[6]. Jarrett et al.[7] demonstrated in the conscious dog that glucagon inhibited contraction of the gall bladder when given prior to cholecystokinin but given alone did not cause relaxation of the gall bladder.

The effect of glucagon on choledochal function was first studied by Lin and Spray[8] who showed in the dog, using a constantly perfused water manometer, that choledochal resistance was lowered. They also described a biphasic effect of glucagon at doses greater than $5 \, mg \, kg^{-1}$ whereby initially there was a rise in resistance followed by a fall[9]. In humans Nebel[10], using a perfused tube inserted into the sphincter of Oddi at the time of ERCP, demonstrated a basal pressure of $32 \pm 4 \, mmHg$ which was reduced by $9 \pm 2 \, mmHg$ after $1 \, mg$ intravenous glucagon. Using a similar technique Geenen et al.[11] described phasic activity of the sphincter of Oddi, the amplitude of which was reduced from $128 \pm 17 \, mmHg$ to $54 \pm 12 \, mmHg$ whilst the phasic activity was reduced from 5.0 ± 0.5 to 1.6 ± 0.6 contractions per minute. The maximal effect of glucagon was seen at 3 minutes, being largely dissipated by 10 minutes.

The action of glucagon on the biliary tree is probably a direct one by increasing the intracellular level of cAMP, as such agents as theophylline and isoproterenol that increase tissue levels of cAMP relax the sphincter in vitro[12]. Propanolol, atropine, phenoxybenazime or pentolinium do not block the effect of glucagon on the biliary tree, suggesting that its action is a direct one[9].

Glucagon also has a choleretic effect, the maximum increase in bile flow of dogs being seen at an infusion rate of $8 \, \mu g \, kg^{-1} \, h^{-1}$ glucagon with no further increase of flow as the dose is increased[13]. In man, Dyck and Janowitz[14] found an increase in bile flow with increasing bolus doses of glucagon until a maximum was reached with a dose of $0.5 \, \mu g \, kg^{-1}$ which had increased bile flow by $155 \pm 14 \%$ of the control value.

In clinical practice glucagon has been studied during biliary radiomanometry and cholangiography, but the results are conflicting. Vinson et al.[15] reported that $10 \, \mu g \, kg^{-1}$ glucagon had abolished spasm of the sphincter of Oddi seen at the time of radiomanometry. The same authors also described a series of 21 patients who received either $4 \, \mu g \, kg^{-1}$ or $10 \, \mu g \, kg^{-1}$ glucagon in 14 of whom it lowered the recorded emptying pressure; flow into the duodenum in 6 only occurred after the glucagon injection. The resting pressure of the common bile duct was lower in 12 patients after glucagon administration[16].

Non-specific obstruction of the distal common bile duct seen during post-operative T-tube or transhepatic cholangiography was abolished completely in 8 out of 12 cases after 1 mg intravenous glucagon[17]. During operative cholangiography glucagon overcame spasm of the sphincter of Oddi seen in 10 patients[18]. A series of 28 patients undergoing post-operative T-tube cholangiograms were given 0.5 mg intravenous glucagon which in 23 improved the demonstration of the choledochoduodenal junction[19].

However, McCarthy[20] reported that in 10 patients given 1 mg glucagon during radiomanometry there was no or only equivocal evidence of relaxation of the sphincter of Oddi.

This work would suggest that glucagon may be useful in the management of painful biliary tract disease, but unfortunately there is only one reported, uncontrolled, trial of the use of glucagon in painful biliary tract disease[22]. This trial consisted of two groups; the first was 31 patients suffering from acute right upper abdominal pain, which was confirmed to be due to cholelithiasis, who received a single injection of 0.2 mg to 1 mg glucagon. 84% of the patients were said to be pain free within 20 seconds to 5 minutes of the injection. In the second group of 71 patients, 61 had had an endoscopic sphincterotomy for choledocholithiasis, 5 had a stone obstructing the cystic duct and 5 had retained common bile duct stones after cholecystectomy. These patients received a loading dose of 1 mg glucagon followed by a continuous infusion of 3–5 mg every 24 hours for between 2 and 12 days. 91% of the patients who had had an endoscopic sphincterotomy and glucagon infusion passed the stones spontaneously, 3 of each of the other two groups successfully resolved with glucagon treatment alone, the other 4 required operative intervention. Results from other centres indicate that 80% of stones will pass after sphincterotomy[23], thus it is difficult to state that any benefit resulted from the use of a glucagon infusion.

An infusion dose of 5 mg h^{-1} glucagon has been reported to have served as a useful therapeutic adjunct in the management of biliary calculi in 6 out of 7 patients[24].

Relaxation of the gall bladder caused by glucagon may allow an impacted stone to dislodge thus allowing free flow of bile and preventing further inflammation. By lowering the resistance of the sphincter of Oddi and increasing bile flow, glucagon should assist the passage of common bile duct calculi into the duodenum.

In Nottingham we are conducting a double blind randomized trial to test the value of pancreatic glucagon in the treatment of painful biliary tract disease. We are now able to present our preliminary results.

All patients on whom a clinical diagnosis of painful biliary tract disease has been made have been entered into the trial after obtaining written informed consent. The patients then received either 1 mg i.v. glucagon bolus followed by 1 mg i.v. every 4 hours for 24 hours as a continuous infusion, or matching placebo. History and examination were recorded on admission and the patients were reviewed at 12, 24 and 36 hours when the examination was repeated. The time at which the patient was pain free was recorded as were all haematological, biochemical and radiological investigations.

To date 50 patients have been entered into the trial, 17 have since been withdrawn as gall stones have not been proven. Of the 33 with proven cholelithiasis, 15 received glucagon and 18 placebo. There were 12 females in the glucagon group, 13 females in the placebo group, and the mean ages of the groups were 54.0 ($\pm$5.11 SEM) years and 56.05 ($\pm$3.48 SEM) years respectively.

On admission there were no statistically significant differences in the distribution of pain, tenderness, guarding or rebound tenderness in the two groups. At 24 hours only 41.7% of the glucagon group complained of pain in the right hypochondrium compared to 92.9% in the placebo group ($X^2 = 5.7$, $p < 0.02$). Patients who received glucagon were pain free at a mean of 12.00 ($+2.99$ SEM) hours and the placebo group 32.11 ($\pm$7.12 SEM) hours (Mann Whitney U, $p < 0.02$). The mean total dose of pethidine given to the glucagon group was 98.33 ($\pm$29.32 SEM) mg, the placebo group 144.22 ($\pm$40.06 SEM) mg, though this difference is not statistically significant.

Abdominal tenderness was graded as being absent, mild, moderate, or severe. Using this system, those patients given glucagon showed a more rapid improvement of tenderness in the right hypochondrium at 12 hours ($X^2 = 7.66$, $p < 0.05$). There appeared to be similar improvement in guarding and rebound tenderness, but these did not reach significance.

The number of days spent in hospital was similar in the two groups. There was no significant difference in the patients' heart rate and temperature between the two groups during the first 48 hours of admission. The white cell count, serum amylase and liver function tests showed no significant differences prior to the glucagon infusion, 10 to 16 hours after the infusion was started, or 12 hours after the infusion was stopped. Blood glucose levels measured at the same times surprisingly also showed no significant difference between those patients receiving glucagon and those receiving placebo.

No serious side effects were encountered; a similar number of patients in both groups complained of nausea and vomiting. A common minor problem was inflammation of the vein used to infuse the glucagon/placebo preparation;

this was only seen when there was not a concurrent saline infusion into the vein. When the vein was used for glucagon/placebo infusion alone 13 of 21 patients developed inflammation. It is probable that this inflammation is due to chemical irritation of the vein.

In this study glucagon has relieved the pain associated with painful biliary tract disease more effectively than placebo, but we have not seen any patients who have had almost instantaneous pain relief as described by Paul[22]. No serious side effects of continuous glucagon infusion have been seen. We are continuing this trial in order to see if the encouraging results seen to date are maintained with larger numbers of patients. On the evidence so far it would appear that glucagon is a useful adjuvant in the management of painful biliary tract disease.

THE ACTION OF GLUCAGON ON THE ESOPHAGUS

Glucagon lowers the resting pressure of the lower esophageal sphincter in conscious humans and also blocks the normally seen pressure increase induced by pentagastrin[25]. Ten patients with achalasia were given $60 \mu g \, kg^{-1}$ glucagon which reduced the resting lower esophageal pressure from 35 (± 3.9 SEM) mmHg to 17 (± 2.3 SEM) mmHg ($p < 0.002$) within three minutes of intravenous injection. This effect was seen to last for about 15 minutes[25]. This effect of glucagon has also been used to treat impaction of a food bolus at the lower esophageal sphincter, with success in half the patients[26].

THE ACTION OF GLUCAGON ON THE SMALL INTESTINE

Since Stunkard et al.[27] in 1955 showed that glucagon abolished gastric 'hunger contractions' there has been increasing interest in the physiological and pharmacological role of glucagon in the gastrointestinal tract. Dotevall and Kock[28] showed that an intravenous injection of 0.25 mg to 1 mg of glucagon inhibited motility of the human jejunum and colon. Motility induced by food, prostigmine and morphine was also inhibited, an effect which was seen within 30 seconds of glucagon injection and lasted 10–15 minutes. Although this effect has been demonstrated in dogs[29], more recently Evans et al.[30], using electrodes and mechanical strain gauges sutured to the serosal surface of the bowel, showed that 1 mg glucagon bolus injection caused stimulation of the canine duodenum, an infusion having the same effect. Fasth and Hulten[31] demonstrated inhibition of gastrointestinal motility in cats as well as a considerable and immediate increase of intestinal blood flow following glucagon injection.

The inhibitory effect of glucagon on gastrointestinal motility is now widely used by radiologists for tubeless hypotonic duodenography[32,33]. Satisfactory stomach, duodenal and small bowel hypotonicity can be obtained using 0.25 mg to 0.5 mg glucagon given intravenously, the larger the dose the longer the period of inhibition[34]. Glucagon has also been used successfully as a premedication for endoscopy of the upper gastrointestinal tract, reducing peristalsis and pyloric reflux[35,36].

We have also conducted a study to assess the quantitative effects of glucagon on fasting gastrointestinal motility patterns. Ten fasted subjects were studied using two linked pressure sensitive radiotelemetry capsules (RTC) positioned 50 cm apart, in the antrum and jejunum, and tuned to separate frequencies[37]. Two phase 111 activity fronts of the migrating myoelectrical complex (MMC)[38] were observed and immediately following the second, 1 mg i.v. glucagon was given. Recordings were continued until two further fronts had been observed.

No detectable change in intraluminal pressure was noted after glucagon as measured by the RTCs.

Following glucagon the mean interval between successive MMCs was significantly reduced.

The control of migrating myoelectrical complexes is not yet understood, but in some way glucagon would appear to act upon this control mechanism.

THE ACTION OF GLUCAGON ON THE LARGE INTESTINE

The action of glucagon on the large bowel is similar. Taylor et al.[39] demonstrated that glucagon inhibited both electrical and mechanical activity recorded from the lower colon and rectum, suggesting that its action is a direct one on the colonic smooth muscle. They also conducted a controlled trial using glucagon during barium enema examination, concluding that it was useful for hypotonic examinations of the colon where spasm was a problem. Unlike the duodenum, there was little difference in the diameter of the colon after glucagon. Chowdhury and Lorber[40] confirmed that glucagon caused inhibition of food or morphine induced motor activity of both the distal colon and rectum. Glucagon has been shown to be uniformly successful in relieving functional spasm of the colon when given as an intramuscular injection 5–8 minutes prior to barium enema examination[41]. It has also been used successfully to aid the reduction of paediatric intussusception at the time of barium enema examination[42].

In a controlled trial Norfleet[43] found glucagon to be of no benefit as a premedication for colonoscopy. Foster et al.[44] found in a controlled trial using glucagon at the time of fiberoptic sigmoidoscopy there was no difference in the distance the instrument was advanced in the glucagon and placebo groups, the time taken for the examination was similar in both groups, as was the patients' estimate of discomfort.

An increase in intracolonic pressure is part of the pathophysiology of diverticular disease[45,46], and the inhibitory action of glucagon led Daniel et al.[47] to conduct a trial using the drug in the treatment of diverticular disease. Twenty consecutive patients presenting with symptoms of acute diverticulitis received intravenous glucagon as their primary treatment. Fourteen patients received an injection of 1 mg glucagon every 4 hours for 36 hours; the remainder received the same quantity by continuous slow pump infusion. The results of the glucagon treated group were compared retrospectively with those of an earlier group of 15 consecutive patients treated conventionally.

The improvement in symptoms in the glucagon treated group was dramatic and considerable. The main symptom of the pain was completely abolished within a mean of 12 hours and palpable abdominal masses had resolved at a mean of 2 days. In the conventionally treated group pain persisted for a mean of 4 days and palpable abdominal masses resolved at a mean of 5 days.

It is possible that glucagon, by relaxing the colon and thus the necks of the diverticula, promotes the drainage of the contents of diverticula into the bowel lumen, thus allowing local inflammation to settle.

We are, in Nottingham, conducting a double blind control trial to evaluate the use of glucagon in acute diverticulitis, but the numbers are as yet too small to report.

References

1. Bromer, W. W., Sinn, L. G. and Behrens, O. K. (1957). The amino acid sequence of glucagon. *J. Am. Chem. Soc.*, **79**, 2807
2. Foa, P. P. (1977). *Glucagon: Its Role in Physiology and Clinical Medicine*. In Foa, P. P., Bajaj, J. S., Foa, N. L. (eds.), p. XXVII (New York: Springer)
3. Jones, P. F. (1973). *Emergency Abdominal Surgery*. (Oxford: Blackwell Scientific)
4. Lin, T. M. (1974). Action of secretin, glucagon, cholecystokinin and endogenously released secretin and cholecystokinin on gall bladder, choledochus and bile flow in dogs. *Fed. Proc.*, **33**, 391
5. Chernish, S. M., Miller, R. E., Rosenak, B. D. and Scholz, N. E. (1972). Effect of glucagon on size of visualized human gall bladder before and after a fat meal. *Gastroenterology*, **62**, 1218

6. Cameron, A. J., Phillips, S. F. and Summerskill, W. H. J. (1969). Effect of cholecystokinin, gastrin, secretin and glucagon on human gall bladder muscle in vitro. *Proc. Soc. Exp. Biol. Med.*, **131**, 149

7. Jarrett, L. N., Foster, G. E., Wright, J. W., Evans, D. F., Bell, D. G. and Hardcastle, J. D. (1980). The effect of feeding and exogenous cholecystokinin on the electrical and mechanical activity of the gall bladder. *Br. J. Surg.*, **68**, 354

8. Lin, T. M. and Spray, G. F. (1969). Effect of pentagastrin, cholecystokinin, caerulein and glucagon on the choledochal resistance and bile flow of conscious dogs. *Gastroenterology*, **56**, 1178

9. Lin, T. M. (1975). Action of gastrointestinal hormones and related peptides on the motor function of the biliary tract. *Gastroenterology*, **69**, 1006

10. Nebel, O. T. (1975). Effect of enteric hormones on the human sphincter of Oddi. *Gastroenterology*, **68**, A105

11. Geenen, J. E., Hogan, W. J., Dodds, W. J., Stewart, E. T. and Arndorfer, R. C. (1980). Intraluminal pressure recording from the human sphincter of Oddi. *Gastroenterology*, **78**, 317

12. Andersson, K. E., Anderson, R., Hedner, P. and Persson, C. G. A. (1972). Effect of cholecystokinin on the level of cyclic AMP and on mechanical activity in the isolated sphincter of Oddi. *Life Sci.*, **11**, 723

13. Jones, R. S., Geist, R. E. and Hall, A. D. (1971). The choleretic effects of glucagon and secretin in the dog. *Gastroenterology*, **60**, 64

14. Dyck, W. P. and Janowitz, H. D. (1971). Effect of glucagon on hepatic bile secretion in man. *Gastroenterology*, **60**, 400

15. Vinson, M.-F., Treffot, M.-J., and Quilichini, F. (1977). Radiomanométrie biliaire: Intérêt du glucagon. *N. Presse Med.*, **6**, 2897

16. Treffot, M.-J., Quilichini, F. and Vinson, M.-F. (1979). Biliary surgery, radiomanometry and glucagon. In Picazo, J. (ed.) *Glucagon in Gastroenterology*, pp. 87–93 (Lancaster: MTP)

17. Ferrucci, J. T., Wittenburg, J., Stone, L. B. and Dreyfuss, J. R. (1976). Hypotonic cholangiography with glucagon. *Radiology*, **118**, 466

18. Bordley, J. and Olson, J. E. (1979). The use of glucagon in operative cholangiography. *Surg. Gynecol. Obstet.*, **149**, 583

19. Cannon, P. and Legge, D. (1979). Glucagon as a hypotonic agent in cholangiography. *Clin. Radiol.*, **30**, 49

20. McCarthy, J. D. (1979). Biliary radiomanometry as an investigative tool in biliary tract disease. In Picazo, J. (ed.) *Glucagon in Gastroenterology*, pp. 95–105 (Lancaster: MTP)

21. Evans, A. F. and Whitehouse, G. H. (1979). The effect of glucagon on infusion cholangiography. *Clin. Radiol.*, **30**, 499

22. Paul, F. (1979). The role of glucagon in the treatment of biliary tract pathology. In Picazo, J. (ed.) *Glucagon in Gastroenterology*, pp. 107–120 (Lancaster: MTP)

23. Safrany, L. (1977). Duodenoscopic sphincterotomy and gall stone removal. *Gastroenterology*, **72**, 338

24. Doman, D. B. and Ginsberg, A. L. (1981). Glucagon infusion therapy for biliary tree stones. *Gastroenterology*, **80**, A91

25. Jennewein, H. M., Waldeck, F., Siewert, R., Weisner, F. and Thimm, R. (1973). The interaction of glucagon and pentagastrin on the lower oesophageal sphincter in man and dog. *Gut*, **14**, 861

26. Ferrucci, J. T. and Long, J. A. (1977). Radiologic treatment of esophageal food impaction using intravenous glucagon. *Radiology*, **125**, 25

27. Stunkard, A. J., van Itallie, T. B. and Reis, B. B. (1955). The mechanism of satiety: Effect of glucagon on gastric hunger contractions in man. *Proc. Soc. Exp. Biol.*, **89**, 258

28. Dotevall, G. and Kock, N. G. (1963). The effect of glucagon on intestinal motility in man. *Gastroenterology*, **45**, 364

29. Necheles, H., Sporn, J. and Walker, L. (1966). Effect of glucagon on gastrointestinal motility. *Am. J. Gastroenterol.*, **45**, 34

30. Evans, D. F., Foster, G. E., Hardcastle, J. D., Johnson, F. and Wright, J. W. (1978). The effect of glucagon on the canine duodenum and small intestine. *Br. J. Pharm.*, **64**, 475P

31. Fasth, S. and Hultén, L. (1971). The effect of glucagon on intestinal motility and blood flow. *Acta Physiol. Scand.*, **83**, 169

32. Chernish, S. M., Miller, R. E., Rosenak, B. D. and Schcolz, N. E. (1972). Hypotonic duodenography with the use of glucagon. *Gastroenterology*, **63**, 392

33. Miller, R. E., Chernish, S. M., Rosenak, B. D. and Rodda, B. E. (1973). Hypotonic duodenography with glucagon. *Radiology*, **108**, 35

34. Miller, R. E., Chernish, S. M., Brunell, R. L. and Rosenak, B. D. (1978). Double blind radiographic study of dose response to intravenous glucagon for hypotonic duodenography. *Radiology*, **127**, 55

35. Melsom, M., Myren, J., Larsen, S. and Moe, A. (1977). Comparison of glucagon and pethidine plus atropine as premedication for peroral endoscopy. *Endoscopy*, **9**, 79

36. Qvigstad, T., Larsen, S. and Myren, J. (1977). Comparison of glucagon, atropine and placebo as premedication for endoscopy of the upper gastrointestinal tract. *Scand. J. Gastroenterol.*, **14**, 231

37. Evans, D. F., Foster, G. E. and Hardcastle, J. D. (1981). Motility patterns of the human antrum and jejunum and their association with sleep: studies using a radiotelemetry system. *Gut*, **22**, A424

38. Carlson, G. M., Bedi, B. S. and Code, C. F. (1972). Mechanism of propagation of intestinal myoelectrical complex. *Am. J. Physiol.*, **222**, 1027

39. Taylor, I., Duthie, H. L., Cumberland, D. C. and Smallwood, R. (1975). Glucagon and the colon. *Gut*, **16**, 973

40. Chowdhury, A. R. and Lorber, S. H. (1977). Effects of glucagon and secretin on food or morphine induced motor activity of the distal colon, rectum and anal sphincter. *Am. J. Dig. Dis.*, **22**, 775

41. Gohel, V. K., Dalinka, M. K. and Coren, G. S. (1975). Hypotonic examination of the colon with glucagon. *Radiology*, **115**, 1

42. Fisher, J. K. and Germann, D. R. (1977). Glucagon aided reduction of intussusception. *Radiology*, **122**, 197

43. Norfleet, R. G. (1979). Premedication for colonoscopy. Randomised double blind study for glucagon v placebo. *Gastrointest. Endosc.*, **24**, 164

44. Foster, G. E., Vellacott, K. D., Balfour, T. W. and Hardcastle J. D. (1981). Outpatient flexible fiberoptic sigmoidoscopy, diagnostic yield and the value of glucagon. *Br. J. Surg.*, **68**, 463

45. Parks, S. and Cornell, A. M. (1969). Motility studies in diverticular disease of the colon. *Gut*, **10**, 534

46. Painter, N. S. and Truelove, S. C. (1964). The intraluminal pressure patterns in diverticulosis of the colon. *Gut*, **5**, 201

47. Daniel, O., Basu, P. K. and Al-Samarrae, H. M. (1974). The use of glucagon in the treatment of acute diverticulitis. *Br. Med. J.*, **3**, 720

Address for correspondence:

Professor J. D. Hardcastle,
Department of Surgery, University Hospital,
Queen's Medical Centre,
Nottingham, Notts. NG7 2UH, UK

DISCUSSION

Miller: Taking your study of the myoelectrical activity first, I do not know how to correlate these data with peristalsis. As I interpret your data, glucagon speeded up peristalsis in the small intestine.

Hardcastle: It shortens the time between successive MMCs, but that does not necessarily mean the speed of peristalsis is increased.

Miller: We have conducted a study, ourselves, using barium sulphate and found that glucagon slowed the rate of transit proportionally to the dose of glucagon given. This was particularly true for the time taken for the barium to reach the caecum. This is the opposite to your data.

Hardcastle: Perhaps we are studying two different entities. The initiation and passage of the MMC may not be related to the rate of peristalsis. There is probably a very complex mechanism initiating an MMC which may be associated with a surge of motilin and a large dose of glucagon may in some way alter this mechanism, thus producing a shorter interval between succeeding MMCs.

Christiansen: Apart from the pathophysiological information you will find in your study on painful biliary tract diseases, would you use glucagon in preference to analgesics in these patients?

Hardcastle: We were rather disappointed during the initial part of this study as we had been expecting a rapid relief of pain as reported by Paul (1979), in Picazo, J. (ed.) *Glucagon in Gastroenterology*, pp. 107–120 (Lancaster: MTP). Also there was no clear cut clinical difference between the two groups. So far all we have shown is that the pain and tenderness improve more rapidly in those patients given glucagon; as yet we have not shown that the subsequent course of the patient is in any way altered. I think we have got to wait until the number of patients in the study is larger before we can say that glucagon has a role to play in the management of painful biliary tract disease.

Vilardell: Did any patients have stones in the common bile duct?

Hardcastle: The group is too small to break into subgroups, but as far as I can remember 2 or 3 patients in each group had stones in the common bile duct.

Vilardell: How do you think glucagon relieves pain?

Hardcastle: Most patients with biliary colic have an obstructed gall bladder; in some way glucagon relieves this more effectively than the placebo.

Diamant: Could you comment on the glucose levels in your study?

Hardcastle: There was no significant difference between the two groups when blood glucose levels were measured 10–16 hours after the infusion had been started. I think this is the effect of a continuous dose of glucagon.

Jaspan: I think this is because large doses of glucagon cause insulin release. This may also explain the differences between your study and Professor Miller's study on intestinal transit. Pharmacological levels of glucagon cause the release of insulin and possibly of motilin and of other gastrointestinal hormones. You may therefore be seeing a secondary hormonal effect.

Hardcastle: Before starting the study on painful biliary tract disease we discussed carefully the dose of glucagon to be given and the general consensus at that time was that we should give a large dose to be certain of showing an effect.

Jaspan: If you were to measure, after a bolus of 1 mg glucagon, all the measurable peptides, I think you would be surprised to find what had been stimulated. Certainly insulin, motilin, growth hormone and other peptides are known to be stimulated by glucagon.

Hardcastle: I accept this and it may well be part of the answer to the shortening of the MMC interval.

Jaspan: I think so too.

9

Fulminant hepatic failure: a review

K. OKUDA

Acute fulminant hepatic failure (FHF) with coma is one of the most frustrating diseases for the physician, the prognosis remaining very poor in spite of numerous attempts at treatment. Fulminant hepatic failure may be defined as a coma syndrome resulting from massive necrosis of liver cells, or following any other cause of sudden and severe impairment of hepatic function. It is characterized by progressive and severe mental changes starting with confusion and often rapidly advancing to stupor, coma and death[1]. Fulminant hepatic failure includes not only fulminant viral hepatitis, but also drug induced hepatitis, Reye's syndrome, fatty liver of pregnancy, and other acute severe liver injuries. In the nomenclature and classification of hepatic diseases established by the International Association for the Study of the Liver[2], acute hepatitides are divided into those with and those without coma, and the term 'fulminant' is used synonymously with 'coma', as this classification is based on aetiology.

Difficulty arises with this definition in differentiating FHF from subacute hepatic failure or subacute hepatitis, which represents an ill-defined, yet distinct entity characterized by less rapidly progressive hepatic failure which starts in a similar setting. One of the solutions would be to set a length of time within which or beyond which signs of hepatic failure develop. At the recent International Workshop on 'Subacute hepatic failure and subacute hepatitis' organized by Dr. B. N. Tandon, New Delhi, India, subacute hepatic failure was defined as persistent or progressive jaundice occurring within eight weeks of the onset of the icteric phase and appearance of ascites, with biochemical evidence of liver cell necrosis, verified histologically by submassive or bridging necrosis.

AETIOLOGY AND INCIDENCE

By far the most common cause of FHF is viral hepatitis. The incidence of FHF following acute viral hepatitis has been estimated to be 0.2 to 1.0 %[3,4], but its frequency among hospitalized patients with acute hepatitis is much higher. In a nation-wide survey made by Takahashi[5] in Japan between 1974 and 1977, FHF was found in 5.76 % of 7036 patients with acute hepatitis admitted to major hospitals. Fulminant hepatitis caused by non-hepatitic viruses such as cytomegalo-[6], Epstein-Barr[7] and herpes simplex[8] virus has been reported, but the large majority of cases are due to primary hepatotrophic viruses. Although the relative frequency of each type of hepatitis virus is not clearly determined, it is now established that any hepatitis virus can cause FHF. In the study of Redeker[9], 6(15%) of 42 HBsAg negative cases of fulminant hepatitis were caused by type A virus. A more recent study in the United States showed that of a total of 188 cases of fulminant hepatitis, A hepatitis accounted for 2 %, A hepatitis accompanied by B hepatitis 2 %, B hepatitis 56 %, non-A, non-B hepatitis 34 %, and drug-induced hepatitis 5 %[10].

Beside viruses, a wide variety of chemical agents may cause FHF[11]. The relative incidence of any specific cause in various reports has depended on geographic locations. For instance, acetaminophen (paracetamol) is an important cause of deaths due to FHF in England[12], whereas in France a relatively common cause is the ingestion of mushroom *Amanita phalloides*[13]. Other hepatotoxic chemicals which cause dose-dependent liver damage include yellow phosphorus, carbon tetrachloride, etc. Hepatic injuries caused by other drugs are unpredictable and not dose-dependent. Halothane hepatitis is well known for its tendency to produce severe liver injury. Isoniazid has claimed a number of deaths in the United States among individuals taking this drug for the prophylaxis of tuberculosis[14]. Co-administration of rifampicin seems to increase isoniazid hepatotoxicity[15]. Intravenous administration of tetracycline in large doses may cause a fatal fatty metamorphosis of the liver, particularly in pregnant women. It accounts for a considerable proportion of the cases of acute fatty liver of pregnancy, a very severe liver disease that occurs near term. Impaired protein synthesis has been suggested as the cause of foamy fatty changes of the hepatocytes which are morphologically distinct from steatosis due to ethanol.

Reye's syndrome is a recently recognized disorder in children, characterized by acutely progressive encephalopathy. It seems to be triggered by viral infections and toxins. Jaundice is mild or absent. Metabolic alterations include increased ammonia and decreased citrulline in serum which mimic those seen in ornithine transcarbamylase deficiency. Although no obvious necrosis of the liver is seen under the light microscope, hepatocytes are foamy with fat droplets, and electronmicroscopically, marked changes of the organelles are evident, such as swelling and distortion of mitochondria[16].

HISTOPATHOLOGY

Fulminant hepatic failure is not necessarily the outcome of massive liver cell necrosis. Liver cell dysfunction may be assessed only from the electronmicroscopic alterations as in Reye's syndrome, or foamy fatty metamorphosis as in fatty liver of pregnancy. Fulminant hepatitis used to be a synonym of acute yellow atrophy or massive hepatic necrosis. However, some of the cases of fulminant hepatitis with a longer survival show less extensive necrosis, and the direct cause of death may be a complication secondary to hepatic failure. Horney and Galambos[17] biopsied the liver in 14 patients with fulminant hepatitis within 2 weeks of onset of coma. The findings were multilobular necrosis in 4, bridging necrosis in 9, and only portal inflammation in 1, with no correlation between histology and duration and grade of coma. Karvountzis et al.[18] studied late liver biopsy in 13 patients who survived severe acute viral hepatitis with coma; most showed no significant liver pathology 4 to 10 months after the disease. In Horney's series, however, 3 out of 9 such patients developed chronic liver disease. A recent nation-wide study made in Japan confirmed the observations made by Karvountzis et al. demonstrating only few patients who subsequently developed a protracted course with mild fluctuations of aminotransferase activities; all of these patients had received blood or plasma as a treatment and non-A, non-B hepatitis seemed to be responsible for the protracted course. Milandri et al.[19] assessed liver cell regeneration by measuring interploid DNA in biopsy liver specimens obtained from patients dying from fulminant hepatitis, and found a level of regeneration similar to that of control patients with ordinary acute hepatitis. They concluded that the rate of liver cell destruction is the major determinant in the prognosis of acute liver failure. In contrast, there is evidence that the protracted course of patients with subacute hepatitis is due to impairment in liver cell regeneration. A protracted clinical course following an ordinary attack of acute hepatitis eventuating in fatal hepatic failure is relatively common among the aged, and, according to the literature, among

Indians with poor nutrition. Peters et al.[20] wrote of such a group of patients as suffering 'Inappropriate Regeneration Syndrome'.

IMMUNOPATHOGENESIS

The exact mechanism by which FHF develops following viral hepatitis is not known. B virus hepatitis in which various serological markers are available, may be a good tool for the study of immunological reactions. There is evidence today that the host factors rather than the dose, virulence or strain of the virus are the main determinants in the subsequent course and outcome of B virus infection. B virus is not directly cytopathic, and the liver damage is the result of immunologic reactions. In fulminant B hepatitis, antibody response seems to be enhanced[21], and the speed of clearance of HBsAg from blood is greatly increased. Appearance of anti-HBs in plasma, which is a late event occurring after the disappearance of HBsAg from blood in ordinary acute B hepatitis, is much accelerated in fulminant hepatitis[22]. It is possible that cell-mediated immunity plays an important role in fulminant hepatitis[23]. HBsAg is not found by immunohistological techniques in liver cells in fulminant hepatitis probably because HBsAg containing hepatocytes are immediately eliminated by cell-mediated immune reactions. Galbraith et al.[24] observed the development of fulminant hepatic failure after the withdrawal of immunosuppressive therapy in three patients with malignancy who had acquired B virus infection during the treatment.

CLINICAL MANIFESTATIONS

Shortly after the initial symptoms of malaise and anorexia, jaundice is noted and then signs of encephalopathy. Aminotransferase activity, whose levels do not necessarily reflect severity of disease, is markedly elevated early in the course, and hyperbilirubinaemia follows. In fulminant hepatitis, the liver size may increase at the height of hepatic necrosis, and then shrink. The changes in liver size and shape can now be followed by computed tomography which often demonstrates irregular distribution of necrosis suggested by low densities. Ascites occurs if the patient survives more than five days[11]. Serum bilirubin, mostly conjugated, is usually elevated above 20 mg/dl, but the relative proportion of unconjugated bilirubin increases with the severity of disease. The important clinical signs at examination include fetor hepaticus and flapping tremor beside the mental disturbances. The neuropsychiatric abnormalities are classified into four grades according to severity[1]. Electroencephalographic alterations occur in association with mental disturbances, progressing from slow waves of high amplitude to paroxysms of bilaterally synchronous delta waves and to the terminal fading of low-voltage activity. Multiple spikes occur during convulsions. There may be transient improvement in electroencephalograms, but this does not signify improvement in the general condition of the patient.

ENCEPHALOPATHY AND CEREBRAL OEDEMA

The cause of acute hepatic coma is multifactorial. The putative toxic metabolites that accumulate in blood have not yet been identified. Elevated ammonia in blood is not the only biochemical abnormality, and increased free fatty acids, mercaptans, phenols, bile acids and bilirubin are all toxic. It has been shown in animals that ammonia, free fatty acids and mercaptans act synergistically[25], and experimentally the dose of one of the three to induce coma is much reduced if combined with one of the others. All free amino acids increase in blood except the branched ones which are decreased[26]. Studies in animals have demonstrated that the aromatic amino acids and tryptophan compete with the branched ones for uptake by the central nervous tissue, and due to these concentration differences, more of the aromatic amino acids cross the blood-brain barrier. The increased entry of the aromatic amino acids, which are precursors of neurotransmitter amines, into the brain may lead to the formation of inhibitory 'false' neurotransmitters, such as octopamine and phenylethanolamine[27], and in fact, these are shown to accumulate in animal models and correlate with the onset of encephalopathy.

The use of branched amino acids in the prevention of encephalopathy in FHF is discouraging, unlike its efficacy in chronic encephalopathy, probably because of the much greater increase of aromatic amino acids[28], and the carrier mediated transport system for them[29]. Recent animal studies have demonstrated that middle molecular size substances may alter permeability of the blood-brain barrier to allow entry of toxic metabolites into the brain and contribute to cerebral oedema[30].

Cerebral oedema frequently develops in FHF. In a series of 92 patients clear cerebral oedema was found at autopsy in 38 %[31]. Since the brain is enclosed in a firm osseous vault, oedema results in increased intracranial pressure, decreased blood perfusion and hence anoxia. The exact stage at which cerebral oedema develops is difficult to determine. Often, the first clinical sign is a sudden respiratory arrest followed by the development of fixed dilated pupils and absent brain stem reflexes. Papilloedema is seldom seen. Williams and his group at King's College Hospital in London are currently using a pressure sensor to monitor intracranial pressure[32]. The pressure rises during haemodialysis, but not markedly. The intravenous administration of mannitol is sometimes effective in alleviating oedema.

RENAL FAILURE AND ELECTROLYTE ABNORMALITIES

Renal dysfunction occurs in 70 % of patients with FHF[33], and renal failure in 43 %[34]. About one half of such patients show 'functional renal failure' characterized by low urinary sodium concentrations, low osmolarity and normal renal histology. In the other half, tubular necrosis occurs which is associated with high concentrations of sodium and isosmolarity of urine, and tubular necrosis. Recent evidence strongly suggests a role of endotoxin which is normally cleared by the Kupffer cells, in the development of renal failure[35]. In severe hepatocellular necrosis when the Kupffer cells are no longer functioning, endotoxin spills over into the systemic circulation. Wilkinson *et al.* have demonstrated endotoxaemia in 14 of 22 patients[36]. The kidney behaves as if there were decreased effective intravascular volume, by failing to clear urea and toxic salts, and decreasing water and salt clearance. Factors precipitating hepatorenal syndrome include sudden diuresis by the use of strong diuretics, removal of large amounts of ascites, gastrointestinal haemorrhage, and manoeuvres leading to sudden decrease of intravascular volume[33].

Alkalosis occurs frequently in FHF. The early alkalosis seems to be metabolic, due to hypokalaemia or to a failure to alkalinize the urine, accumulation of basic metabolites and movement of proton into intracellular space. Hyperventilation which develops in the early phase of coma leads to respiratory alkalosis. It is associated with impaired oxygen dissociation from haemoglobin, and reduced perfusion and diminished oxygen consumption in the brain, contributing to the worsening of the neuropsychiatric condition of the patient. Hyponatraemia is also common along with hypokalaemia. It is due in part to haemodilution as a result of renal failure to excrete water, and also to a shift of sodium from plasma into intracellular compartments, an increase of sodium concentration in leucocytes recently having been demonstrated[37].

COAGULOPATHY AND BLEEDING DIATHESIS

Decrease in platelet count, prothrombin level, and concentrations of fibrinogen, factors II, V, VII, IX and X, are the constant abnormalities in FHF. Deficiency in the clotting factors is attributed to reduced synthesis by the liver, but it may also be due to intravascular coagulation as suggested by thrombocytopenia in the absence of megakaryocyte abnormality in the marrow, accelerated plasma disappearance of labelled fibrinogen, and the presence of fibrin-degradation products in plasma[11]. Gastrointestinal bleeding occurs in more than 50% of patients. Bleeding is often from gastric erosions, and the acidity of gastric juice seems to be the important factor. Bleeding may be prevented by keeping pH above 5[38], but this is difficult[39], and recent studies have advocated the use of H_2-receptor antagonists[32]. Bleeding into extra-gastrointestinal organs also occurs, but haemorrhage is not always the leading cause of death[4,40]. The frequency with which haemorrhage proves to be the direct cause of death varies with the report. Whereas in Rueff's series it was the direct cause of death in only 5 of 60 patients, an incidence of 11 out of 30 was given in the series of Williams[31], and in Saunders's series life-threatening haemorrhage occurred in more than half the adult patients and in 70% of the children[41].

OTHER COMPLICATIONS

Pulmonary oedema is another complication common in FHF which has not received much attention. According to Trewby et al.[42], 37 out of 100 consecutive patients with FHF had clinical and radiological evidence of pulmonary oedema. However, none had clinical signs of left heart failure while pulmonary artery wedge pressure was normal. There was a certain correlation between cerebral and pulmonary oedema, suggesting a common factor or a central nervous origin of pulmonary oedema. Structurally, the major abnormality is a diffuse dilatation of the pulmonary vascular bed affecting arteries and veins of all structural types[43]. Thus, respiratory failure is perhaps due to a number of factors. Although the patient responds to positive end-expiratory pressure ventilation, positive pressure ventilation theoretically produces potential difficulties in liver diseases. Due to the downward pressure of the diaphragm, hepatic vein pressure increases up to 60%, decreases blood flow out of the liver, and aggravates ischaemic necrosis of centrilobular zones. With increased tidal volume, the splanchnic circulation, including the portal blood flow, decreases, adding further to the vicious circle of the event[33].

Infection and the septicaemia that will follow can also be life-threatening events. It is frequently the respiratory and urinary tracts that are affected. Ascites which is common in FHF has generally been attributed to hypoalbuminaemia. Recent evidence obtained from the measurement of hepatic vein pressures in fulminant hepatitis suggests that the gradient between free and wedge pressures is increased in patients with ascites; this is perhaps due to massive necrosis[44].

MANAGEMENT

The mortality in FHF is between 80 and 90 % in adults, though survival occurs more frequently in younger age groups[11]. In the past, corticosteroids were used without supporting data in the management of FHF. Recent controlled trials in the use of corticosteroids have failed to show improved survival over controls[45,46]. In animal models, however, administration of steroids very early in the development of signs of hepatic failure suggests that this may be beneficial[47]. It may act by tightening the blood-brain barrier, thus preventing an increase in permeability[48]. Exchange transfusion, extracorporeal animal liver perfusion, cross circulation with a human being or baboon, and plasmapheresis are based on the rationale of removing toxic metabolites which accumulate in blood, in order to allow liver cells to regenerate before the liver fails totally. The conscious level of the patient often improves temporarily when these procedures are carried out, but few eventually survive. Several animal model studies have demonstrated the capability of charcoal columns to remove water soluble toxic substances, and have encouraged charcoal haemoperfusion as an artificial liver support. In an early trial of charcoal in the treatment of FHF at King's College Hospital in London a 37.8 % survival rate was obtained[49]. However, subsequent studies by the same group have failed to repeat this result, probably due to changes in the biocompatibility and quality of charcoal; many patients succumbed to uncontrollable hypotension after the use of charcoal. It soon became clear that platelet aggregates formed during the passage of blood through the charcoal[50], and release of vasoactive amines caused hypotension. To avoid such difficulties, prostacyclin, which protects platelets both *in vitro* and *in vivo*, has recently been used with some success[51]. The surface of the charcoal has been improved by various coating techniques to minimize physical effects on formed blood elements. Separation of plasma in the haemoperfusion system before making contact with charcoal is another way of avoiding the adverse effects of charcoal.

Following the difficulties associated with charcoal haemoperfusion, attempts were made to develop a haemodialysis system to remove toxic substances. Instead of cuprophan membrane, Opolon used the Rhône–Poulenc system with polyacrylnitrite membrane which is highly permeable permitting removal of middle molecular size substances of up to 5000[52]. It has a significant effect in improving the conscious level of the patient, but its eventual effect on survival has yet to be determined. A recent figure on survival at King's College Hospital among 108 patients with FHF treated with such a haemodialysis system was 28.7 %[32]. Patients with paracetamol-induced FHF seemed to respond better than those with fulminant hepatitis. There is evidence that protein-bound toxins also increase in FHF and need to be removed. To that end, resins of the Amberlite series seem to be effective[53], but biocompatibility of the resin has to be improved in order to fit in the liver support system. Artificial liver support systems have yet to be developed and tested, and at the moment the prospect of such developments occurring is uncertain. Some sort of liver transplant, when the diagnosis is made early, may be developed in the future. In the meantime, conservative but vigorous medical management is most important[54]. Administration of insulin-glucagon to accelerate regeneration of hepatocytes may be beneficial when the patient has sustained the initial fulminant attack. A recent collaborative study in Japan[5] clearly demonstrated the presence of two separable groups of patients with fulminant hepatitis, the acute group developing coma within ten days of onset and the other subacute group later. The prognosis was much poorer in the subacute group, most spontaneous recoveries occurring in the acute group.

References

1. Trey, C. G. and Davidson, C. S. (1970). The management of fulminant hepatic failure. In Popper, H. and Schaffer, F. (eds.) *Progress in Liver Disease*, Vol. 3, p. 282 (New York: Grune and Stratton)
2. Diseases of the Liver and Biliary Tract. Standardization of Nomenclature, Diagnostic Criteria, and Diagnostic Methodology. Fogarty International Center Proc. No. 22. (1977). DHEW Publication No. (NIH) 77-725, Washington, D.C., 1
3. Lucke, B. and Mallory, T. (1946). The fulminant form of epidemic hepatitis. *Am. J. Pathol.*, 22, 867
4. Boughton, C. R. (1968). Viral hepatitis in Sydney: a review of fatal illnesses in a hospital series. *Med. J. Aust.*, 2, 343
5. Takahashi, Y., Shimizu, M. and Kosaka, M. (1979). Nationwide statistics of severe hepatitis (fulminant hepatitis). (In Japanese) *Saishin Igaku*, 34, 2285
6. Henson, D. E., Crimley, P. M. and Strano, A. J. (1974). Postnatal cytomegalovirus hepatitis: an autopsy and liver biopsy study. *Hum. Pathol.*, 5, 93
7. Chang, M. Y. and Campbell, W. G., Jr. (1975). Fatal infectious mononucleosis: association with liver necrosis and herpes-like virus particles. *Arch. Pathol.*, 99, 185
8. Connor, R. W., Lorts, S. and Gilbert, D. N. (1979). Lethal herpes simplex virus type 1 hepatitis in a normal adult. *Gastroenterology*, 76, 590
9. Redeker, A. G. (1978). Advances in clinical aspects of acute and chronic liver disease of viral origin. In Vyas, G. N., Cohen, S. N. and Schmid, R. (eds.) *Viral Hepatitis. A Contemporary Assessment of Etiology, Epidemiology, Pathogenesis and Prevention*, p. 425 (Philadelphia: Franklin)
10. Acute Hepatic Failure Study Group represented by Rakela, J. (1979). Etiology and prognosis in fulminant hepatitis. *Gastroenterology*, 78, A33
11. Rueff, B. and Benhamou, J.-P. (1973). Acute hepatic necrosis and fulminant hepatic failure. *Gut.* 14, 805

12. Sherlock. S. (1979). Hepatic reactions to drugs. *Gut*, **20**, 634

13. Sicot, C., Bismuth, C., Pebay-Peyroula, F., Frejaville, J. P. and Rueff, B. (1969). Eléments du pronostic des intoxications phalloidiennes. *J. Eur. Toxicol.* **2**, 250

14. Garibaldi, R. A., Drusin, R. E., Ferebee, S. H. and Gregg, M. B. (1972). Isoniazid-associated hepatitis: report of an outbreak. *Am. Rev. Resp. Dis.*, **106**, 357

15. Passayre, D., Bentata, M., Degott, C., Nouel, O., Mguet, J.-P., Rueff, B. and Benhamou, J.-P. (1977). Isoniazid-Rifampsin fulminant hepatitis. A possible consequence of the enhancement of isoniazid hepatotoxicity by enzyme induction. *Gastroenterology*, **72**, 284

16. Schubert, W. K., Partin, J. C. and Partin, J. S. (1972). Encephalopathy and fatty liver (Reye's syndrome). In Popper, H. and Schaffner, F. (eds.) *Progress in Liver Disease*, Vol. 4, p. 489 (New York: Grune and Stratton)

17. Horney, J. T. and Galambos, J. T. (1977). The liver during and after fulminant hepatitis. *Gastroenterology*, **73**, 639

18. Karvountzis, G. G., Redeker, A. G. and Peters, R. L. (1974). Long term follow-up studies of patients surviving fulminant viral hepatitis. *Gastroenterology*, **67**, 870

19. Milandri, M., Gaub, J. and Ranek, L. (1980). Evidence for liver cell proliferation during fatal acute liver failure. *Gut*, **21**, 423

20. Peters, R. L., Omata, M., Aschavai, M. and Liew, C. T. (1978). Protracted viral hepatitis with impaired regeneration. In Vyas, G. N., Cohen, S. N. and Schmid, R. (eds.) *Viral Hepatitis. A Contemporary Assessment of Etiology, Epidemiology, Pathogenesis and Prevention*, p. 79 (Philadelphia: Franklin)

21. Trepo, C. G., Robert, D., Motin, J., Sepetijian, M. and Prince, A. M. (1976). Hepatitis B antigen (HBsAg) and or antibodies (anti-HBs and anti-HBc) in fulminant hepatitis: pathogenic and prognostic significance. *Gut*, **17**, 10

22. Woolf, I., El Sheikh, N., Cullens, H., Lee, W. M., Eddleston, A. L. W. F., Williams, R. and Zuckerman, A. J. (1976). Enhanced HBsAg production in pathogenesis of fulminant viral hepatitis type B. *Br. Med. J.*, **2**, 669

23. Dudley, F. J., Fox, R. A. and Sherlock, S. (1972). Cellular immunity in hepatitis associated Australia antigen disease. *Lancet*, **1**, 723

24. Galbraith, R. M., Eddleston, A. L. W. F., Williams, R., Zuckerman, A. J. and Bagshawe, K. D. (1975). Fulminant hepatic failure in leukaemia and choriocarcinoma related to withdrawal of cytotoxic drug therapy. *Lancet*, **2**, 528

25. Zieve, L., Doizaki, W. M., and Zieve, F. J. (1974). Synergism between mercaptans and ammonia or fatty acids in the production of coma: a possible role for mercaptans in the pathogenesis of hepatic coma. *J. Lab. Clin. Med.*, **83**, 16

26. Fisher, J. E. and Baldessarini, R. J. (1976). Pathogenesis and therapy of hepatic coma. In Popper, H. and Schaffner, F. (eds.) *Progress in Liver Disease*, Vol. 5, p. 363 (New York: Grune and Stratton)

27. Fisher, J. E., Funovics, J. M., Aguirre, A., James, J. H., Kerne, J. M., Wesdorp, R. C. C., Yoshimura, N. and Westman, T. (1974). Plasma amino acids in patients with hepatic encephalopathy. *Am. J. Surg.*, **127**, 40

28. Rosen, M. M., Yoshimura, N., Jodgman, J. M. and Fisher, J. E. (1977). Plasma amino acid pattern in hepatic encephalopathy of differing etiology. *Gastroenterology*. **72**, 483

29. Partridge, W. A. and Oldendorf, W. H. (1973). Kinetic analysis of blood-brain barrier transport of amino acid. *Bioch. Biophys. Acta*, **401**, 128

30. Bloch, P., Delorme, M. L., Rapin, J. R., Goschat, M. and Opolon, P. (1978). Reversible modifications of brain neurotransmitters in experimental acute hepatic coma. *Surg. Obstet. Gynecol.*, **146**, 551

31. Williams, R. (1972). Hepatic failure and development of artificial liver support system. In Popper, H. and Schaffner, F. (eds.) *Progress in Liver Disease*, Vol. 4, p. 418 (New York: Grune and Stratton)

32. Jenkins, P. J. and Williams, R. (1980). Fulminant viral hepatitis. *Clin. Gastroenterol.*, **9**, 171

33. Rogers, E. L. and Rogers, M. C. (1980). Fulminant hepatic failure and hepatic encephalopathy. *Pediatr. Clin. N. Am.*, **27**, 701

34. Wilkinson, S. P., Moodie, H., Arroyo, V. A. and Williams, R. (1977). Frequency of renal impairment in paracetamol overdose compared with other causes of acute liver damage. *J. Clin. Path.*, **30**, 141

35. Liehr, H., Grün, M. and Brunswig, D. (1976). Endotoxemia in acute hepatic failure. *Acta Hepato-Gastroenterol.*, **23**, 235

36. Wilkinson, S. P., Arroyo, V., Gazzard, B. G., Moodie, H. and Williams, R. (1974). Relation of renal impairment and haemorrhagic diathesis to endotoxaemia in fulminant hepatic failure. *Lancet*, **1**, 521

37. Alam, A. N., Wilkinson, S. P., Poston, L., Moodie, H. and Williams, R. (1977). Intracellular electrolyte abnormalities in fulminant hepatic failure. *Gastroenterology*, **72**, 914

38. Opolon, P. and Caroli, J. (1974). Etudes des facteurs du traitement des atrophies hépatiques aiguës d'origine virale. *J. Méd. Intern.*, **121**, 1

39. MacDougall, B. R. D., Bailey, R. J. and Williams, R. (1977). H_2-receptor antagonists and antacids in the prevention of acute gastrointestinal haemorrhage in fulminant hepatic failure. *Lancet*, **1**, 617

40. Ritt, D. J., Whelan, G., Werner, D. J., Eigenbrodt, E. H., Schenker, S. and Combes, B. (1969). Acute hepatic necrosis with stupor or coma: an analysis of thirty-one patients. *Medicine*, **48**, 151

41. Saunders, S. J., Hickman, R., MacDonald, R. and Terblanche, J. (1972). The treatment of acute-liver failure. In Popper, H. and Schaffner, F. (eds.) *Progress in Liver Disease*, Vol. 4, p. 333 (New York: Grune and Stratton)

42. Trewby, P. N., Warren, R., Contini, S., Crosbie, W. A., Wilkinson, S. P., Laws, J. W. and Williams, R. (1978). Incidence and pathophysiology of pulmonary edema in fulminant hepatic failure. *Gastroenterology*, **74**, 859

43. Williams, A., Trewby, P., Williams, R. and Reid, L. (1979). Structural alterations to the pulmonary circulation in fulminant hepatic failure. *Thorax*, **34**, 447

44. Lebrec, D., Nouel, O., Bernuau, J., Rueff, B. and Benhamou, J.-P. (1980). Portal hypertension in fulminant viral hepatitis. *Gut*, **21**, 962

45. Gregory, P. B., Knauer, C. M., Kempson, R. L. and Miller, R. (1976). Steroid therapy in severe viral hepatitis. *N. Engl. J. Med.*, **294**, 681

46. Redeker, A. G., Schweitzer, I. L. and Yamahiro, H. S. (1976). Randomization of corticosteroid therapy in fulminant hepatitis. *N. Engl. J. Med.*, **294**, 728

47. Hanid, M. A., MacKenzie, R. L., Jenner, R. D., Chase, R. A., Mellon, P. J., Trewby, P. N., Janota, I., Davis, M., Silk, D. B. A. and Williams, R. (1979). Intracranial pressure in pigs with surgically induced liver failure. *Gastroenterology*, **76**, 123

48. Rovit, R. L. and Hagan, R. (1978). Steroids and brain oedema: the effects of glucocorticoids on abnormal capillary permeability following cerebral injury in cats. *J. Neuropathol. Exp. Neurol.*, **27**, 277

49. Gazzard, B. G., Weston, M. J. and Murray-Lyon, I. M. (1975). Experience at King's College Hospital with charcoal haemoperfusion: overall results in 37 patients. In Williams, R. and Murray-Lyon, I. (eds.) *Artificial Liver Support*, p. 234 (London: Pitman)

50. Langley, P. G., Hughes, R. D., Ton, H. Y., Davies, M., Hanid, M. A., Mellon, P. J., Silk, D. B. A. and Williams, R. (1978). Further studies on the blood compatibility of polyhemacoated charcoal in haemoperfusion systems. *Proc. Eur. Soc. Artif. Org.*, **5**, 142

51. Gimson, A. E. S., Langley, P. G., Hughes, R. D., Canales, J., Mellon, P. J., Williams, R., Woods, H. F. and Weston, M. J. (1980). Prostacyclin to prevent platelet activation during charcoal haemoperfusion in fulminant hepatic failure. *Lancet*, **1**, 173

52. Opolon, P., Lavallard, M., Crubille, C., Gateau, P., Nusinoviv, V., Granger, A., Darnis, F. and Caroli, J. (1975). Encéphalopathie au cours de l'atrophie hépatique aiguë. Effet de l'eparation des moyennes molecules. Résultats preliminaires. *Nouv. Presse Méd.*, **4**, 2987

53. Willson, R. A. (1975). Resins as adsorbents — including experimental studies in dogs with obstructive jaundice. In Williams, R. and Murray-Lyon, I. (eds.) *Artificial Liver Support*, p. 109 (London: Pitman)
54. Auslander, M. O. and Gitnick, G. L. (1977). Vigorous medical management of acute fulminant hepatitis. *Arch. Intern. Med.*, **137**, 599

Address for correspondence

Professor K. Okuda,
Professor of Medicine,
First Department of Medicine,
Chiba University Medical School,
1-8-1 Inohana,
Chiba City (280),
Japan

DISCUSSION

Baker: This is a very interesting review, Professor Okuda. I should like to ask a question regarding the Japanese study you mentioned. Did that study produce any data correlating the likelihood of death with the histology of the liver? Personally I do not know of any good studies on this syndrome in which the degree of liver damage has correlated with the likelihood of death. The studies you mentioned by American investigators were follow up studies performed a number of months later.

Okuda: At a meeting in Gifu, in, I believe, June of this year, Dr. Takahashi of Gifu University asked if any clinicians had had the opportunity to follow patients surviving an acute attack of fulminant hepatitis. There were a number of cases where histology was available. The data were shown in a poster session, and although the conclusions have not yet been published, the clinicians' impressions were that some cases would eventually develop into hepatitis. But all of these patients had had blood transfusion or plasma exchange, so it is now felt that they may have had a non-A, non-B, rather than chronic hepatitis sequelae after the initial attack.

Baker: I take the point you made in your lecture well about the impaired regeneration syndrome and the possible usefulness of insulin and glucagon for treatment of this group of patients. It seems to me also that in patients with the more common type of fulminant hepatic failure, even though there are studies to suggest that regenerative activity may be normal, there is such extensive cell necrosis that if regeneration can be stimulated some of those patients might survive who now expire, particularly if the likelihood of dying is related to the degree of cell necrosis.

Jaspan: Professor Okuda, your comments about the encephalopathy were well taken. I find them very interesting and I should like to ask you a question related to this. A concern that I have is in the use of glucagon in high doses, because Soeters and co-workers have suggested that encephalopathy may be due to the B branched chain amino acids being reduced, resulting in decreased competition for entry into brain such that tryptophan and other aromatic amines are transported into brain, where they are converted into serotonin and perhaps other neurotransmitters with potentially important adverse effects (Soeters, P. *et al.* (1975). *Gastroenterology*, **69**, A-67, 867). As you mentioned, there has been correlation between encephalopathy and some amino acid levels, and the concern I have is in using very high levels of glucagon, which may be appropriate pharmacologically but which may aggravate the amino acid disturbance. As you well know, if you look at liver failure patients and particularly those with portacaval shunts, the glucagon levels are bordering on pharmacologic levels. They can be 10-, 15-, 20-fold elevated. Do you have any data to suggest that encephalopathy may worsen in patients receiving glucagon infusion?

Okuda: Not at the moment, I am afraid.

Baker: Let me ask one other question about the background information that you presented. What is the latest information on the mechanism of brain oedema and cerebral permeability? Is it the middle molecules that produce that? Is there any good data in humans?

Okuda: At the present moment we know very little about the mechanism of brain oedema, or of what it means.

10

Aspects of hormonal influence on liver growth

N. L. R. BUCHER, W. E. RUSSELL and J. A. McGOWAN

WHOLE ANIMAL STUDIES

The continuing research for the mechanisms that control growth and regeneration of the liver was reviewed by Volpicelli[1] at the first workshop in this series in 1978, and subsequently by ourselves and others in 1979 and 1980[2-4]. Salient points from this large body of research are briefly considered here to delineate outstanding problems as perspectives for current work.

First, as is well known, adult liver parenchymal cells are normally quiescent, but possess an impressive latent growth potential, as evidenced by the intense burst of proliferative activity following acute liver loss or injury.

Second, this proliferative activity is under humoral control as demonstrated by numerous liver transplant and cross circulation experiments[5,6].

Third, portal venous blood is enriched with humoral agents – so-called hepatotrophic factors – that can promote liver growth; in addition to nutrients, these include insulin, glucagon, and possibly other factors. The evidence, which is extensive, is based upon liver transplants supplied with portal compared to systemic blood, and on complex rearrangements of hepatic circulation coupled with ablation of various portal splanchnic organs[1,2,4-6].

Fourth, insulin and glucagon are not primary initiators of liver growth, and do not significantly stimulate multiplication of liver cells when infused into normal animals; rather, they seem to serve permissive or modulating roles[5,7,8].

Fifth, epidermal growth factor (EGF), especially in combination with insulin or glucagon, does initiate liver growth in normal animals[6,9]; other hormonal mixtures involving triiodothyronine (T_3) or catecholamines and also containing glucagon are likewise effective[10,11].

Sixth, in addition to the foregoing, liver growth can be induced or modulated experimentally by manipulation of diet and feeding schedules.

The evidence implies that insulin, glucagon, EGF, and certain other known hormones and nutrients regulate liver growth, and that unknown humoral agents – so-called hepatotrophic factors – do likewise; whether these unknown humoral agents include some or all of the known substances mentioned, or others, remains conjectural.

(a) Insulin

Studies of a number of kinds of cells in culture carried out in serum free media point to insulin as a nearly universal requirement for growth[12], and its function in potentiating liver growth is well established[1-4]. Under at least some conditions, very low concentrations of insulin seem able to support active liver growth; liver regenerated at near normal rates in partially hepatectomized rats made diabetic with alloxan (as evidenced by ^{3}H-labelling of DNA[13]), and at 15–20% of normal rates in rats acutely deprived of pancreatic and gastrointestinal hormones by portal splanchnic evisceration[14]. Probably minimal insulin concentrations were present in the diabetic animals, and intracellular hormonal influences may have persisted in the evisceration experiments in which blood insulin was near or below limits of detection by radioimmunoassay. Furthermore, in normal animals whose livers regenerate actively following partial hepatectomy, portal venous insulin levels were observed to fall abruptly[15,16], and the rate of regeneration was not augmented by insulin administration. Further reduction of the already low insulin levels in these partially hepatectomized rats by infusion of anti-insulin serum, however, significantly depressed DNA synthesis, underscoring the role of insulin in potentiating the growth process[6].

Under some conditions, low levels of insulin do not suffice; high doses were necessary to provide maximal enhancement of EGF-stimulated DNA synthesis and mitosis in normal intact livers[6,9]. Whether in these instances insulin is performing a somatomedin-like or other role in addition to its usual functions, or whether the cells are more resistant to its actions under certain conditions is unsettled. It appears that insulin is essential for full expression of liver growth, and the requisite concentration varies somewhat with circumstances; lower than normal levels, however, can support even the highest proliferative activity.

(b) Glucagon

There is far less of a consensus regarding the role of glucagon[1,2,4,6,7,17-20]. In the portal splanchnic eviscerated, partially hepatectomized rats, previously referred to, infusion of high doses of insulin and glucagon together dramatically restored the depressed rates of liver regeneration to normal; each hormone by itself was ineffective[7,8]. This is consonant with the prior studies of Price and his associates who emphasized the role of glucagon but overlooked the importance of the striking synergistic interaction of the two hormones, because in their experiments insulin was continuously present[21,22]. On the contrary, Starzl and his co-workers found that in dogs neither insulin nor glucagon, separately or in combination, was able to stimulate the depression of hepatic regeneration resulting from portal splanchnic evisceration[17,23]. The divergent findings probably arise from differences in species and experimental conditions; current studies, discussed later, suggest that the metabolic state of the livers at the time the combined insulin-glucagon treatment is instituted may be determinative.

The effectiveness of the insulin-glucagon treatment in the evisceration experiments described depended upon physiologic doses of insulin, but pharmacologic doses of glucagon. Pharmacologic glucagon dosage was likewise required in the EGF-plus-glucagon and other hepatic growth-inducing hormonal mixtures (e.g. T_3, amino acids, heparin, and glucagon (the TAGH formula) devised by Short et al.[10], and catecholamines-plus-glucagon devised by Hasegawa and Koga[11]). In a different experimental model we observed that insulin and pharmacologic doses of glucagon strikingly increased survival of mice lethally infected with A-59 murine hepatitis virus[20,24]. It remains unclear why these exceedingly high doses of glucagon are required, and whether or not its action upon the liver under these various circumstances is secondary to effects exerted elsewhere in the body.

As insulin and glucagon are involved with protein and amino acid metabolism, and as hepatocyte proliferation can be induced by subjection of rats for several days to a protein free diet followed by an amino acid meal[25], we examined the effects of this dietary treatment upon portal venous insulin and glucagon levels[16]. Following partial hepatectomy insulin levels fell and glucagon concentration rose; in the protein depleted-refed rats, changes in these hormone levels followed a similar course, as did those in animals starved for 2–3 days and then refed amino acids. The latter animals, however, showed no elevation of DNA synthesis. Reproduction of the endogenous patterns of portal venous insulin and glucagon concentrations associated with partial hepatectomy or amino acid depletion and repletion is therefore not by itself sufficient to induce liver growth. This is consistent with the evidence that these two hormones may facilitate but not initiate liver growth.

(c) Epidermal growth factor

The possible hepatotrophic role of EGF is of particular interest, because as noted, unlike insulin and glucagon it can initiate hepatocyte proliferation in the quiescent, intact livers of normal adult rats[6,9]. EGF, which is a 53 amino acid single chain polypeptide similar in molecular weight to insulin, is a broad spectrum mitogen, stimulating wound healing and proliferation of epithelial cells *in vivo*, and growth of many cell types from numerous species in culture[26,27]. The blood level, which in the mouse is 1 ng/ml, rises over 100-fold upon stimulation with phenylephrine. The hormone urogastrone, isolated from human urine, appears to be the human form of EGF; it is found in extracts of the submandibular salivary gland, thyroid, duodenum, jejunum, and kidney, but the concentrations are very low (about 1–6 ng/g wet tissue), and it is not certain that these tissues are the only sources of the relatively large amount appearing in the urine (about 50 μg/day)[28]. This large amount is remarkable in view of its 1.5 minute half-life in the serum; possibly it circulates as a prehormone that can undergo proteolytic activation in areas of required action[27]. In addition to its mitogenic action EGF is a potent inhibitor of gastric acid secretion; its major physiologic role remains unclear.

Somewhat like insulin, the concentration of EGF in the circulation appears to fall within an hour after partial hepatectomy in rats[3].

Recently St. Hilaire *et al.* have found that normal liver sequesters I^{125}-labelled EGF from the blood and secretes it, along with breakdown products, into the bile; this observation suggests a role for the liver in maintaining EGF homeostasis[29]. Earp[30] has determined that binding of I^{125}-EGF by liver cell membranes decreases as early as 8 hours following partial hepatectomy, reaching a nadir at 36–48 hours; this decrease is attributable to the well established 'down regulation' of EGF receptor number that attends cellular stimulation by EGF. (When EGF binds to its receptor on the cell surface the EGF-receptor complex is internalized and the number of available receptors is thereby decreased.) The authors tentatively conclude that this EGF binding to receptors has a physiologic role in the complex response to partial hepatectomy.

This brief discussion of results from whole animal studies illustrates the inherent difficulties. Despite knowledge of specific substances capable of inducing and modulating liver growth, the actual blood components exerting physiologic control remain conjectural; many problems remain, including the central one of precisely how these hormonal agents, which are effective mitogens in many types of cells, can limit stimulation only to liver under conditions of hepatic deficiency, leaving other organs unaffected.

A major impediment to further progress has been that the liver cells within the animal are always subject to unknown influences from other organs, so that direct effects of experimental variables cannot be reliably ascertained.

PRIMARY HEPATOCYTE MONOLAYER CULTURES

An alternative approach is through cell culture, in which, despite an artificial environment, growth signals can be examined singly and in combinations, and mechanisms of action sought without intrusion of extraneous influences. A new dimension has been added to cell culture research by the work of Sato and his associates[12], demonstrating that the requirement of cell cultures for serum can be met by various combinations of hormones and growth factors, nutrients, and other known compounds, so that many types of cells can now be grown in chemically defined media; an important finding is that each type of cell requires its own particular combination of these substances for the full expression of growth and differentiated functions. One or more key combinations of factors could therefore deliver a specific signal to one particular type of cell.

Application of these principles to the problem of control of liver growth has gained impetus from the development of a workable methodology for isolation and culture of adult hepatocytes[31,32], and from the observation that although these hepatocytes do not actively proliferate in culture[33–38], they can be stimulated to synthesize DNA, which is an essential early step in the proliferative sequence[39]. This permits scrutiny of the important early events and the factors that control them as the cells undergo the transition from quiescence (G_0/G_1 phase) to the 'S phase' (i.e., DNA synthesis). This is the segment of the cell cycle where physiologic controls are generally considered to operate. It should thus become possible to re-examine critically the concepts that have so far emerged from the studies in whole animals.

In quest of hepatotrophic serum factors, we are currently studying the effects of hormones, growth factors and serum components in short-term primary monolayer cultures of adult rat hepatocytes. The hepatocytes are freshly isolated from young adult male rats by perfusion of the liver with buffered collagenase solution[32,40]. The isolated cells are maintained in culture

145

for three days in a serum free, chemically defined medium (Waymouth's MAB 87/3), modified to promote hepatocyte survival and suppress growth of unwanted cells. For assessment of DNA synthesis, ^{3}H-thymidine is added for the final 24 hours, and the DNA is then extracted and assayed for radioactivity[40]. These cultures are virtually free of cells other than hepatic parenchymal cells.

Although the cells will survive for considerably longer than three days, they are reported to develop characteristics of fetal liver[36,41–43], and we therefore believe that short-term primary cultures should reflect physiologic states of the adult liver more closely than cells adapted to extraneous influences in artificial media for prolonged periods.

(a) Epidermal growth factor and insulin

Under the conditions employed, the hepatocytes respond to the presence of EGF in the culture medium with a rise in ^{3}H-thymidine incorporation into DNA which is maximal at 48–72 hours. Insulin, only slightly stimulatory by itself, synergistically augments the EGF stimulation, elevating the incorporation many-fold above that in unsupplemented medium[39,40]. This is similar to *in vivo* observations, mentioned earlier, and shows unequivocally that these two hormonal agents exert their effects directly upon the hepatocytes without mediation by other kinds of cells or their products.

(b) Rat serum

In view of the extensive evidence mentioned earlier, that humoral signals control liver growth, we have begun to study rat serum[44]. The results show that normal rat serum, dialysed to eliminate nutrients and other small molecular components, is not only several times more effective in stimulating DNA synthesis than a variety of sera from other species including human, mouse, rabbit, equine and bovine (fetal, newborn, and calf) sera, but is also more potent than EGF plus insulin. Serum collected from rats at numerous intervals after partial hepatectomy, however, so far fails to exceed normal serum. This is contrary to the evidence from the whole animal studies.

We are now investigating numerous possible explanations for this divergence, and attempting to fractionate rat serum to determine what the active components may be. We find that more than half of the stimulatory activity of both normal and partially hepatectomized rat sera is derived from the blood platelets. As various substances can accrue to blood platelets[45], it is not certain where in the body the platelet factor originates. We have partially purified rat platelet lysate by gel filtration and ion exchange chromatography, and so far have only observed a single peak of activity, with a molecular weight of about $75\,000$[46]. Human serum also contains a platelet-derived growth factor, termed PDGF, which has been purified and well characterized[47]. It differs from the rat platelet factor in several respects including molecular size and heat stability, and it so far fails to stimulate rat hepatocyte cultures, although it effectively potentiates growth of a number of cell types from several species. We have not yet examined rat platelet factor activity derived from partially hepatectomized animals.

(c) Glucagon

Meanwhile we are also studying effects of glucagon which by itself, as *in vivo*, fails to cause more than minimal stimulation of hepatocyte cultures. In our initial investigation glucagon consistently augmented the stimulus provided to the cultures by the EGF-insulin mixture, and this could be reproduced by replacement of the glucagon with dibutyryl-cyclic AMP or any of several substances such as isoproterenol, cholera toxin, or isobutylmethylxanthine, that are known to elevate intracellular cyclic AMP concentrations[40]. This is in agreement with the known mediation of other actions of glucagon by cyclic AMP.

For further clarification of the roles of insulin and glucagon, we have recently begun to explore the interactions of these two hormones and several nutrients in the medium. Although stimulation of DNA synthesis with EGF, and further enhancement by combination with insulin, remained highly reproducible regardless of changes in the 'energy substrates' in the medium, the addition of glucagon or dibutyryl-cyclic AMP under these conditions yielded paradoxical effects, sometimes causing a rise and sometimes a fall in DNA biosynthetic activity. It appears from preliminary studies that under certain experimental conditions in the presence of EGF supplemented with insulin and glucose, addition of glucagon leads to further enhancement of DNA synthesis, as observed in the initial investigation[40]. Addition of pyruvate to the EGF-insulin mixture also enhances the stimulus; on the other hand, if glucagon is added when high concentrations of pyruvate are present, the glucagon then becomes ineffective or inhibitory. This reversal of glucagon action seems to be less pronounced when insulin or glucose levels are lowered. Other components of the system, including hydrocortisone which is routinely present, have not been adequately explored, and no clear explanation for the paradoxical behaviour of glucagon can yet be offered. At present, we merely wish to emphasize the complexity of the interactions, and our emerging view that the effects of glucagon may change radically depending upon the metabolic state of the cell. Eventually these studies should account for the divergent results obtained with glucagon in the evisceration experiments discussed earlier. It is clear that glucagon, like EGF and insulin, exerts its growth promoting effects through direct action upon the hepatocytes; whether the huge doses required for effectiveness *in vivo* depend in addition upon ancillary actions of other affected organs, or an overwhelming of some hepatocytic function, or other cause, has not yet been determined.

SUMMARY

In summary, the physiological control of regeneration and growth of adult liver, on the basis of whole animal studies extending over many years, appears to reside in blood borne substances. Among these may be insulin, glucagon, EGF, other hormonal factors, and nutrients. EGF modestly stimulates DNA synthesis; it is synergistically augmented by insulin and glucagon which seem to have facilitating or modulating roles in the growth process. Hepatic growth signals are complex, and the extent of involvement of these and other substances remains to be settled.

In primary monolayer hepatocyte cultures, sera from normal or partially hepatectomized rats stimulate DNA synthesis with equal potency. This is at variance with *in vivo* evidence, which supports enhanced hepatotrophic activity in the blood during hepatic regeneration. Over half of the *in vitro* stimulatory activity of normal rat serum resides in a polypeptide (molecular weight about 75 000) derived from the blood platelets. The rat platelet factor seems to differ from human PDGF, and is being further characterized.

EGF, insulin, and glucagon affect hepatocytes directly, without intervention of other cell types; in cultures, as *in vivo*, EGF stimulates DNA synthesis, and is greatly enhanced by insulin. Glucagon (or cyclic AMP) still further augments this stimulation under some conditions; under others it is ineffective or inhibitory. Preliminary data suggest that this reversal of glucagon action may depend upon the presence of certain 'energy substrates', and the metabolic state of the cells.

The demonstration of synergistic interactions among hormonal agents supports the likelihood of a multifaceted control mechanism. Growth signals may be modulated by seemingly minor changes in key hormone concentrations.

Acknowledgement

This work was supported by USPHS Grants Nos. CA02146 and AM19435.

References

1. Volpicelli, N. A. (1979). Hepatotrophic effects of insulin and glucagon and their potential role in the treatment of hepatic failure. In Picazo, J. (ed.) *Glucagon in Gastroenterology*, pp. 121–130 (Lancaster: MTP Press)

2. Bucher, N. L. R. and McGowan, J. A. (1979). Regeneration: regulatory mechanisms. In Wright, R., Alberti, K. G. M. M., Karran, S. and Millward-Sadler, G. (eds.) *Liver and Biliary Disease*, pp. 210–227 (London: W. B. Saunders)

3. Leffert, H. L., Koch, K. S., Moran, T. and Rubalcava, B. (1979). Hormonal control of rat liver regeneration. *Gastroenterology*, **76**, 1470

4. Starzl, T. E. (1980). The ripple effect of liver transplantation. *Transplant. Proc.*, **12**, 626

5. Hays, D. M. (1974). Surgical research aspects of hepatic regeneration. *Surg. Gynecol. Obstet.*, **139**, 609

6. Bucher, N. L. R., Patel, U. and Cohen, S. (1978). Hormonal factors concerned with liver regeneration. In CIBA Foundation Symp. #55 *Hepatotrophic Factors*, pp. 95–107 (Amsterdam: Excerpta Medica)

7. Bucher, N. L. R. and Swaffield, M. N. (1975). Regulation of hepatic regeneration in rats by synergistic action of insulin and glucagon. *Proc. Natl. Acad. Sci. USA*, **72**, 1157

8. Bucher, N. L. R. and Swaffield, M. N. (1975). Synergistic action of glucagon and insulin in relation to hepatic regeneration. In Weber, G. (ed.) *Advances in Enzyme Regulation*. Vol. 13, pp. 281–293 (New York: Pergamon)

9. Bucher, N. L. R., Patel, U. and Cohen, S. (1978). Hormonal factors and liver growth. In Weber, G. (ed.) *Advances in Enzyme Regulation*. Vol. 16, pp. 205–213 (New York: Pergamon)

10. Short, J., Brown, R. F., Husakova, A., Gilbertson, J. R., Zemel, R. and Lieberman, I. (1972). Induction of deoxyribonucleic acid synthesis in the liver of the intact animal. *J. Biol. Chem.*, **247**, 1757

11. Hasegawa, K. and Koga, M. (1977). Induction of liver cell proliferation in intact rats by amines and glucagon. *Life Sci.*, **21**, 1723

12. Barnes, D. and Sato, G. (1980). Methods for growth of cultured cells in serum-free medium. *Analyt. Biochem.*, **102**, 255

13. Younger, L. R., King, J. and Steiner, J. F. (1966). Hepatic proliferative response to insulin in severe alloxan diabetes. *Cancer Res.*, **26**, 1408

14. Bucher, N. L. R. and Swaffield, M. N. (1973). Regeneration of liver in rats in the absence of portal splanchnic organs or portal blood supply. *Cancer Res.*, **33**, 3189

15. Bucher, N. L. R. and Weir, G. C. (1976). Insulin, glucagon, liver regeneration, and DNA synthesis. *Metabolism*, **25**, 1423

16. Bucher, N. L. R., McGowan, J. A. and Patel, U. (1978). Hormonal regulation of liver growth. In Dirksen, E. R., Prescott, D. M. and Fox, C. F. (eds.) *ICN-UCLA Symposia on Molecular and Cellular Biology*. Vol. XII, pp. 661–670 (New York: Academic Press)

17. Starzl, T. E., Francavilla, A., Porter, K. A., Benichou, J. and Jones, A. F. (1978). The effect of splanchnic viscera removal upon canine liver regeneration. *Surg. Gynecol. Obstet.*, **147**, 193

18. Starzl, T. E., Porter, K. A., Kashiwagi, N. and Putnam, C. W. (1975). Portal hepatotrophic factors, diabetes mellitus and acute liver atrophy, hypertrophy and regeneration. *Surg. Gynecol. Obstet.*, **141**, 843

19. Starzl, T. E., Porter, K. A., Watanabe, K. and Putnam, C. W. (1976). Effects of insulin, glucagon, and insulin/glucagon infusions on liver morphology and cell division after complete portacaval shunt in dogs. *Lancet*, **1**, 821

20. Farivar, M., Wands, J. R., Isselbacher, K. J. and Bucher, N. L. R. (1976). Effect of pancreatic hormones on fulminant murine hepatitis. *N. Engl. J. Med.*, **295**, 1517

21. Whittemore, A. D., Kasuya, A., Voorhees, A. B., Jr., and Price, J. B., Jr. (1975). Hepatic regeneration in the absence of portal viscera. *Surgery*, **77**, 419

22. Price, J. B., Jr. (1976). Insulin and glucagon as modifiers of DNA synthesis in the regenerating rat liver. *Metabolism*, **25** (suppl. 1), 1427

23. Starzl, T. E., Francavilla, A., Porter, K. A. and Benichou, J. (1978). The effect upon the liver of evisceration with or without hormone replacement. *Surg. Gynecol. Obstet.*, **146**, 524

24. Bucher, N. L. R. (1977). In Weber, G. (ed.) *Advances in Enzyme Regulation*. Vol. 15, pp. 221–230 (New York: Pergamon)

25. Short, J., Armstrong, N. B., Kolitsky, M. A., Mitchell, R. A., Zemel, R. and Lieberman, I. (1974). In Clarkson, B. and Baserga, R. (eds.) *Control of Proliferation in Animal Cells*, pp. 37–48 (New York: Cold Spring Harbor Laboratory)

26. Carpenter, G. and Cohen, S. (1979). Epidermal growth factor. *Ann. Rev. Biochem.*, **48**, 193

27. Hollenberg, M. D. (1979). EGF-urogastrone, a polypeptide acquiring hormonal status. *Vitam. Horm.* **37**, 69

28. Hirata, Y. and Orth, D. N. (1979). Epidermal growth factor (urogastrone) in human tissues. *J. Clin. Endocrinol. Metab.*, **48**, 667

29. St. Hilaire, R. J., Jones, A. L., Hradek, G. T. and Kim, Y. S. (1981). A quantitative electron microscopic and biochemical analysis of hepatic uptake and processing of epidermal growth factor (EGF). *Gastroenterology*, **80**, 1347

30. Earp, H. S. and O'Keefe, E. J. (1981). Epidermal growth factor receptor number decreases during rat liver regeneration. *J. Clin. Invest.*, **67**, 1580

31. Berry, M. N. and Friend, D. S. (1969). High yield preparation of isolated rat liver parenchymal cells. A biochemical and fine structural study. *J. Cell Biol.*, **43**, 506

32. Seglen, P. O. (1976). Preparation of isolated rat liver cells. In Prescott, D. M. (ed.) *Methods in Cell Biology*, pp. 29–83 (New York: Academic Press)

33. Laishes, B. A. and Williams, G. M. (1976). Conditions affecting primary cell cultures of functional adult rat hepatocytes. II. Dexamethasone enhanced longevity and maintenance of morphology. *In Vitro*, **12**, 821

34. Wanson, J. C., Drochmans, P., Mosselmans, R. and Ronveaux, M.-F. (1977). Adult rat hepatocytes in primary monolayer culture. *J. Cell Biol.*, **74**, 858

35. Seglen, P. O., Solheim, A., Grinde, B., Gordo, P., Schwarze, P., Gjessing, R. and Poli, A. (1980). Amino acid control of protein synthesis and degradation in isolated rat hepatocytes. *Ann. N.Y. Acad. Sci.*, **349**, 1

36. Ichihara, A., Nakamura, T., Tanaka, K., Tomita, Y., Aoyama, K., Sato, S. and Shinno, H. (1980). Biochemical function of adult rat hepatocytes in primary culture. *Ann. N.Y. Acad. Sci.*, **349**, 77

37. Sirica, A. E. and Pitot, H. C. (1980). Drug metabolism and effects of carcinogens in cultured hepatic cells. *Pharm. Rev.*, **31**, 205

38. Grisham, J. W. (1980). Cell types in long term propagable cultures of rat liver. *Ann. N.Y. Acad. Sci.*, **349**, 128

39. Richman, R. A., Claus, T. H., Pilkis, S. J. and Friedman, D. L. (1976). Hormonal stimulation of DNA synthesis in primary cultures of adult rat hepatocytes. *Proc. Natl. Acad. Sci. USA*, **73**, 3589

40. McGowan, J. A., Strain, A. J. and Bucher, N. L. R. (1981). DNA synthesis in primary cultures of adult rat hepatocytes in a defined medium: effects of epidermal growth factor, insulin, glucagon and cyclic-AMP. *J. Cell. Physiol.*, **108**, 353

41. Leffert, H. L., Moran, T., Sell, S., Skelly, H., Ibsen, K., Mueller, M. and Arias, I. (1978). Growth state-dependent phenotypes of adult hepatocytes in primary monolayer cultures. *Proc. Natl. Acad. Sci. USA*, **75**, 1834

42. Sirica, A. E., Richards, W., Tsukada, Y., Sattler, C. A. and Pitot, H. C. (1979). Fetal phenotypic expression by adult rat hepatocytes on collagen gel/nylon meshes. *Proc. Natl. Acad. Sci. USA*, **76**, 283

43. Guguen-Guillouzo, C., Szajnert, M.-F., Glaise, D., Gregori, C. and Schapira, F. (1981). Isoenzyme differentiation of aldolase and pyruvate kinase in fetal, regenerating,

preneoplastic and malignant rat hepatocytes during culture. *In Vitro*, **17**, 369

44. Strain, A. J., McGowan, J. A. and Bucher, N. L. R. (1981). Stimulation of DNA synthesis in primary cultures of adult rat hepatocytes by rat platelet-associated substance(s). *In Vitro*, **18**, 108

45. Adelson, E. A., Rheingold, J. J. and Crosby, W. H. (1961). The platelet as a sponge: a review. *Blood*, **17**, 767

46. Russell, W. E. and Bucher, N. L. R. (1981). Hepatotrophic peptide from rat platelets. *J. Cell Biol.*, **91**, 204a

47. Scher, C. D., Shepard, R. C., Antoniades, H. N. and Stiles, C. D. (1979). Platelet-derived growth factor and the regulation of the mammalian fibroblast cell cycle. *Biochim. Biophys. Acta*, **560**, 217

Address for correspondence

Dr. N. L. R. Bucher,
Associate Professor of Surgery (Oncology),
Harvard Medical School,
Massachusetts General Hospital,
Shriners Burns Institute,
51 Blossom Street,
Boston, MA 02114,
USA

DISCUSSION

Baker: It is clear that glucagon has a multitude of actions, but could you, I wonder, speculate on the mechanism of its effect on DNA? Is it a membrane effect, an energy substrate effect, or what?

Bucher: We *think* that it may have something to do with the kind of substrates that are being metabolized, but this is pure speculation as we do not have definite information at present.

Jaspan: Do you think it might have something to do with the receptors?

Bucher: Perhaps. When isolating cells we attempt to minimize damage to the receptors, although this is difficult to evaluate. The hepatocytes seem to respond more slowly to hormones in culture than they do *in vivo*, possibly because they may need a 'recovery period' for restoration of receptors.

Jaspan: Leffert and many others have looked at this question (Leffert, H. *et al.* (1975). *Proc. Natl. Acad. Sci. U.S.A.*, **72**, 4033; Leffert, H. and Kock. K. S. (1978). In Ciba Foundation Symposium 55 *Hepatotrophic Factors*, pp. 61–94. New York: Elsevier, Excerpta Medica, North Holland). I know that glucagon receptors and insulin receptors are very much affected by nutritional status in animals.

Bucher: What we intend to do eventually is to treat animals *in vivo* in ways that will influence the receptors, to find out whether the effects are subsequently reflected in the behaviour of the cells in culture.

Jaspan: I noticed one very important difference between your *in vivo* and your *in vitro* studies, and that was that insulin rather than EGF was dominant *in vivo*, whereas it is jut the reverse *in vitro*.

Bucher: I would not put too much weight on that. The results probably depend upon relative amounts of insulin, glucagon and EGF, as well as the prior metabolic state of the cells. The scope of the *in vivo* studies was restricted by the limited availability of EGF. Its halftime in the blood stream is very short – only about 8 minutes (Cohen, S. and Savage, R. C. (1974). *Recent Prog. Horm. Res.*, **30**, 551) – so that relatively large amounts are required. We did not have access to enough to do a thorough study on hormone dosage permutations.

Oriol Bosch: I think your data make sense when one considers that glucagon's acute effect may have something to do primarily with utilizing energy for the secretion of glucose, while a secondary effect is the synthesis of DNA. What one could be observing by adding glucagon is, since what you are measuring is the synthesis of DNA, a shifting of priorities towards the secretory action on the hepatocyte. One therefore sees this lowering of DNA synthesis, which perhaps is only the result of the available energetic resources being used for another priority. This is only an hypothesis, but it could explain these apparently contradictory data.

Bucher: Possibly. I should point out, however, that the art of culturing adult hepatocytes is not yet fully developed. The cells do not survive indefinitely, and although they can undergo a round of DNA synthesis, they do not actively proliferate.

In the animal, on the other hand, when the cell has committed itself to synthesize DNA it then progresses through mitosis to finish the cycle. The cultures may be lacking in certain essential conditions or factors. Perhaps under certain conditions glucagon can make up for some of these deficiencies. EGF appears to be an important motivating force for inducing DNA synthesis, as it is also effective *in vivo* (Bucher, N. L. R., *et al.* (1978). In Ciba Foundation Symposium 55 *Hepatotrophic Factors*, pp. 95–109. New York: Elsevier, Excerpta Medica, North Holland), but it is not unique in this regard. *In vivo* the hepatocytes are proliferatively quiescent; one sees about 1 mitosis per 20 000 cells. These quiescent cells are partially activated, however, merely by being isolated and placed in culture, because a limited number enter DNA synthesis even when no hormone or growth factors are added. This could be due to perturbation of the cell surface by exposure to enzymes, or other aspects of the cell isolation procedure, or to down-shifts or up-shifts of critical nutriments, or other unknown influences. This aspect of the culture system requires further study.

11

Insulin and glucagon for liver disease: assessment of response in patients with alcoholic hepatitis

A. L. BAKER

INTRODUCTION

Recent animal investigations suggest that hepatotrophic factors are present in portal venous blood and contribute to liver regeneration following hepatic injury. Thus, Marchioro *et al.* demonstrated that canine liver segments maintained with portal venous flow show strikingly greater hyperplasia when compared with controls perfused with peripheral venous flow[1]. Blood returning to the liver from the pancreatic-duodenal bed is more effective in stimulating liver hyperplasia than blood from the lower splanchnic circulation[2]. In addition, Starzl *et al.* showed that atrophy of the left hepatic lobe of the dog can be prevented after portacaval shunting by infusion of insulin into the corresponding portal vein[3]. In these studies glucagon alone had no effect and did not potentiate the beneficial effect of insulin[3]. However, Bucher *et al.* found that both insulin and glucagon are required for maximal hepatic regeneration in eviscerated rats subjected to partial hepatectomy[4]. Also, Farivar *et al.* demonstrated that mortality is reduced and liver injury lessened in mice infected with murine A-59 hepatitis virus only when both insulin and glucagon are administered[5]. Insulin and glucagon were both necessary not only for improvement in mortality but also for stimulation of radioactive thymidine incorporation and repair of hepatic histology. These studies suggest important but not necessarily exclusive roles for both insulin and glucagon in the control of hepatic regeneration in mammals.

Because these observations suggested that insulin and glucagon might offer a new approach to treatment of liver injury in humans, we undertook a randomized controlled trial to test this hypothesis in alcoholic hepatitis. Patients with this disease were chosen for study because the mortality of alcoholic hepatitis is as high as 65% in some series recently published for university medical centres[6–9] and because of the frequency of the disease.

METHODS

(a) Selection and treatment of patients

This study was designed to select patients with alcoholic hepatitis varying widely in severity, since this treatment had not been previously investigated in this disease and it was not known which patients were likely to respond. The study was also designed to assess mortality, the clearest end-point in a clinical trial involving patients with a disease of high mortality. In addition, standard liver function tests were performed at regular intervals throughout study, as well as several unique tests of liver function, including the aminopyrine breath test (ABT), alpha fetoprotein, and amino acid profiles.

The admission records of all patients hospitalized in the medical services of the University of Chicago Medical Center between 1st October 1976 and 1st December 1978 were reviewed for evidence of alcoholic hepatitis. All patients admitted with a presumptive diagnosis of alcoholic hepatitis were considered to be candidates for this study. The diagnosis was based on the following criteria: a history of alcohol consumption of 120 g or more per day for more than one year or a history of multiple repetitive alcohol binges for years, or family substantiation of prolonged excessive alcohol consumption without specific quantitation. A liver biopsy demonstrating the lesion of alcoholic hepatitis was also required, unless prolongation of the prothrombin time refractory to parenteral vitamin K_1 precluded biopsy. When a biopsy could not be performed, the SGOT was required to be abnormal and greater than the SGPT. Patients with serious infections, gastrointestinal bleeding, or pancreatitis were excluded from study.

Histologic alcoholic hepatitis was recognized by the presence of an inflammatory hepatic lesion with hydropic cells, centrilobular hepatocellular necrosis, and polymorphonuclear leukocytic infiltration. Mallory's alcoholic hyalin, although supportive of the diagnosis, was not required. Fifty-one of the 82 patients who fulfilled the criteria for entry into the study agreed to participate. These patients gave fully informed written consent to a protocol meeting the Guidelines of the Declaration of Helsinki and approved by the University of Chicago Clinical Investigation Committee.

Twenty-six patients were assigned to insulin and glucagon treatment and 25 to control infusion using sealed envelopes and computer generated random numbers. The treated patients received regular insulin 2 U/h and glucagon 200 µg/h in 200 ml 5 % dextrose in water via a peripheral vein over 12 h daily for three weeks. Control group patients received 5 % dextrose according to a similar schedule. Two grams of human serum albumin were added to the bottles containing insulin and glucagon to prevent adsorption of the hormones to the infusion apparatus and to the control bottles to maintain identical appearance of the solutions.

(b) Assessment of response

Clinical features of liver disease including ascites, spider angiomas, hepatic and splenic enlargement, and severity of encephalopathy were determined and recorded for each patient on admission to the study and at weekly intervals thereafter. Liver function tests including total serum bilirubin, SGOT, SGPT, alkaline phosphatase, albumin, globulin, and prothrombin time were performed on admission to the study and thereafter weekly. Fasting blood specimens for measurement of insulin and glucagon levels were also drawn on admission. At weekly intervals thereafter blood specimens were taken for measurement of insulin and glucagon levels 3 to 4 h after breakfast with the infusions running. Radioimmunoassays of these hormones were performed utilizing previously described methods[10,11]. Each patient was also studied with barium radiographs or endoscopy to determine whether esophageal varices were present.

To assess liver function dynamically all patients also received an ABT, a non-invasive measurement of hepatic microsomal enzyme function[12], on entry into the study and at weekly intervals. Amino acid profiles were measured in 21 patients (10 insulin and glucagon and 11 control), and the branched chain to aromatic amino acid ratio was determined as previously described[13,14]. Alpha fetoprotein, an oncofetal protein which may reflect hepatic regeneration[15], was measured in 20 patients (10 insulin and glucagon and 10 control) at the beginning and end of the study. All patients were admitted to the general medical or gastroenterology services, and most patients were transferred to the Clinical Research Center for completion of the investigations following initial improvement in the hospital. When caloric intake seemed inadequate, nutritional supplements were prescribed. Unless special diets were indicated because of the presence of hepatic encephalopathy or ascites, patients received a 2200 calorie diet.

RESULTS

(a) Patients investigated

Only one of the fifty-one patients who met the criteria for admission failed to complete the study. This patient, who was assigned to insulin and glucagon treatment, left the hospital against medical advice on the second day of study, and is not included in the data analysis. All surviving patients completed 21 days of treatment. The demographic features and clinical characteristics of liver disease and mean values for liver function tests were similar in the two groups at the time of entry into the study, except for a somewhat higher SGOT in the control group (Tables 1 and 2).

(b) Survival and complications

Nine (18 %) of the 50 patients died during the study; six of these underwent autopsy and the diagnosis of alcoholic hepatitis was confirmed in all. Three (12 %) of 25 patients in the insulin and glucagon group, and 6 (24 %) of 25 patients in the control group died (Table 3, $p < 0.24$, Fisher exact test). The

Table 1 Patients studied

	Insulin and glucagon group ($n = 25$)	Control group ($n = 25$)
Female	9 (36%)	12 (48%)
Male	16 (64%)	13 (52%)
Black	23 (92%)	17 (68%)
White	2 (8%)	8 (32%)
Mean age (years ± SD)	44 ± 10	41 ± 9
Liver biopsy	7 (28%)	9 (36%)
Number of days hospitalized before entry into study (mean ± SD)	6.3 ± 4.3	5.1 ± 2.8

(Baker, A. L. *et al.*, 1981. Reprinted, with permission, from *Gastroenterology*, **80**, 1410)

158

Table 2   Clinical and biochemical features of disease at time of entry into study

	Insulin and glucagon group (n = 25)	Control group (n = 25)
Varices	14 (56%)	9 (36%)
Hepatomegaly > 12 cm	21 (84%)	17 (68%)
Splenomegaly	10 (40%)	9 (36%)
Fever > 38 °C	8 (32%)	4 (16%)
Spider angiomas	5 (20%)	6 (24%)
Encephalopathy	10 (40%)	9 (36%)
Ascites	15 (60%)	16 (64%)
Total bilirubin (mg/dl)*	9.0 ± 8.4	11.8 ± 10.7
Prothrombin time (s)*	16.3 ± 2.2	16.5 ± 2.7
Albumin (g/dl)*	2.4 ± 0.4	2.5 ± 0.5
SGOT (IU)*	81 ± 28	$122 \pm 76, p < 0.05$
SGPT (IU)*	34 ± 18	44 ± 32
Alkaline phosphatase (IU)*	104 ± 47	97 ± 56
Venous ammonia (mg/dl)*	225 ± 135	245 ± 165

* = Mean $\pm$ SD

(Baker, A. L. et al., 1981. Reprinted, with permission, from Gastroenterology, **80**, 1410)

cause of death in the 6 control patients and in 2 of the 3 insulin and glucagon treated patients was hepatic failure. Serious infections, gastrointestinal haemorrhage, or the hepatorenal syndrome developed in these patients. The other death in the insulin and glucagon infused group was related to

Table 3   Characteristics upon entry into the study of patients who died during its course

	Insulin and glucagon group	Control group	p value
Total patients studied	25 (50%)	25 (50%)	
Total deaths	3 (12%)	6 (24%)	<0.25
Liver failure	2	6	
Hypoglycaemia	1	0	
Number patients with total bilirubin > 6.0 mg/dl and prothrombin time > 3 s prolonged	9	12	
Deaths	1 (11%)	5 (41%)	<0.15
Number patients with prothrombin time > 3 s prolonged	15	19	
Deaths	1 (7%)	6 (32%)	<0.10

(Baker, A. L. et al., 1981. Reprinted, with permission, from Gastroenterology, **80**, 1410)

hypoglycaemia resulting from the combined effects of decreased food intake, severe liver disease, and the insulin infusion. Two other insulin and glucagon infused patients also developed hypoglycaemia but responded to infusion of 50% dextrose and were maintained in the study without further complication. Because of possible hypoglycaemia, all subsequent patients had frequent blood sugar measurements performed on venous blood by the hospital clinical laboratory or on finger stick blood specimens by Dextrostix®. Macular skin eruptions developed in three patients but did not resemble findings described in association with glucagonomas. These patients were treated symptomatically and continued on infusion therapy.

To determine which patients might respond better to insulin and glucagon therapy, patients were stratified as to disease severity after the study code was broken. Mortality was less in the insulin and glucagon treated patients with a total bilirubin greater than 6.0 mg/dl and a prothrombin time greater than 3 s prolonged (Table 3, $p < 0.15$, Fisher exact test). Mortality was also less in the 15 insulin and glucagon treated patients with prothrombin times greater than 3 s prolonged, but again the difference did not reach statistical significance (Table 3, $p < 0.10$, Fisher exact test).

(c) Laboratory data

The total serum bilirubin levels and prothrombin times showed statistically significant improvements in the insulin and glucagon infused patients ($p < 0.05$, Table 4), whereas the other liver function tests were unchanged. Also, the clinical features of liver disease recorded in this study showed no significant change after three weeks of therapy. In three patients restudied as crossovers during a second episode of alcoholic hepatitis, there were no differences in the standard liver function tests (Table 5). The ABT improved in all surviving patients, and the rate of improvement was somewhat greater in the insulin and glucagon treated patients (Figure 1). However, the difference between the two groups fell just short of statistical significance during the third week of study. There was no improvement in the branched chain to aromatic amino acid ratios in the study patients (Table 6). Also, none of the patients studied with alpha fetoprotein measurements had values above 20 ng/ml, levels occasionally found in apparently normal individuals[15].

Mean plasma insulin and glucagon levels were similar in the two groups before the infusions were begun but increased progressively during the course of the study (Table 7). The significant elevation of both hormones in the insulin and glucagon infused group suggests that the liver was exposed to increased levels of both hormones.

Table 4 Liver function tests in control and in insulin and glucagon treated patients

Test	Results Mean ± SEM			p value
	Baseline	After 3 wks	Absolute change	
Serum bilirubin (mg/dl)				
Control	11.8 ± 1.6	9.3 ± 1.0	− 1.1 ± 1.6	<0.05
Insulin and glucagon	9.0 ± 1.2	4.0 ± 0.7	− 4.3 ± 1.2	
Prothrombin time (s)				
Control	16.5 ± 0.4	16.1 ± 0.6	0.03 ± 0.5	<0.05
Insulin and glucagon	16.3 ± 0.3	14.5 ± 0.3	− 1.5 ± 0.3	
SGOT (IU)				
Control	122 ± 1	69 ± 15	− 19 ± 18	NS
Insulin and glucagon	81 ± 4	108 ± 12	34 ± 11	
SGPT (IU)				
Control	44 ± 5	51 ± 9	6 ± 1	NS
Insulin and glucagon	34 ± 3	76 ± 11	43 ± 9	
Alkaline phosphatase (IU)				
Control	97 ± 8	80 ± 6	− 11 ± 5	NS
Insulin and glucagon	104 ± 7	88 ± 5	− 8 ± 6	
Albumin (g/dl)				
Control	2.5 ± 0.1	3.0 ± 0.2	1.5 ± 0.6	NS
Insulin and glucagon	2.4 ± 0.3	2.8 ± 0.1	1.3 ± 0.4	
Globulin (g/dl)				
Control	4.4 ± 0.8	5.0 ± 0.8	0.8 ± 0.2	NS
Insulin and glucagon	4.4 ± 0.9	4.9 ± 0.8	0.5 ± 0.2	

(Baker, A. L. *et al.*, 1981. Reprinted, with permission, from *Gastroenterology*, **80**, 1410)

DISCUSSION

The present studies suggest that insulin and glucagon may be beneficial for patients with alcoholic hepatitis. Although much interest has focused on new treatments directed specifically at the liver in this disease, particularly using corticosteroids, no clear benefit to treated patients has been established[9,16-20]. We are continuing to study treatment of alcoholic hepatitis with infusion of insulin and glucagon in our institution, hoping that a clearly beneficial effect of this treatment can be demonstrated. These studies are now directed to patients who have the most abnormal liver function tests and thus carry the gravest prognosis. In the present study the trend towards improvement was more apparent in patients where the total serum bilirubin was greater than 6.0 mg/dl and the prothrombin time greater than 3 s prolonged (Table 3, $p < 0.15$, Fisher exact test). The insulin and glucagon treated patients in the 34 subjects with prothrombin times greater than 3 s prolonged also had a lower

Table 5 Crossover data

Patient and order of therapy	Before insulin and glucagon (Entry)				After insulin and glucagon (Week 3)				Before placebo (Entry)				After placebo (Week 3)			
	Serum bilirubin (mg%)	Protime (s)	Serum albumin (g)	SGOT (IU)	Serum bilirubin (mg%)	Protime (s)	Serum albumin (g)	SGOT (IU)	Serum bilirubin (mg%)	Protime (s)	Serum albumin (g)	SGOT (IU)	Serum bilirubin (mg%)	Protime (s)	Serum albumin (g)	SgOT (IU)
~9 (drug first)	13.3	14.5	2.5	138	3.0	13.6	3.0	94	24	18.1	3.9	93	13.2	15.0	2.6	117
~16 (placebo first)	4.8	15.0	2.5	99	3.3	16.1	3.0	210	4.8	17.2	2.4	110	2.5	15.6	2.9	61
~27 (drug first)	20.3	15.7	2.7	91	18.5	15.6	3.5	202	21.2	17.9	2.6	179	13.6	17.9	3.5	116
~32 (placebo first)	20.6	20.3	2.0	74	14.0	15.4	2.7	106	23.6	16.9	2.2	65	13.5	17.2	3.3	106
~55 (placebo first)	3.3	17.9	3.0	129	2.0	17.1	2.6	108	3.1	17.5	2.9	129	2.3	17.0	2.9	108
~56 (drug first)	2.2	12.9	2.5	90	1.3	13.6	3.0	120	3.7	16.6	2.6	134	1.6	14.6	3.1	37

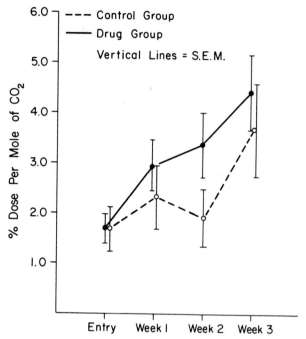

Figure 1 Mean aminopyrine breath test results performed at weekly intervals

Table 6 Branched chain to aromatic amino acid ratios in control and in insulin and glucagon treated patients (mean ± SD)

	Baseline	After 3 weeks	p value*
Control (11)	1.3 ± 0.8	2.1 ± 1.2	NS
Insulin and glucagon (10)	1.5 ± 0.8	1.9 ± 1.0	NS
p value	NS	NS	

Numbers in parentheses = number of patients in each group
* Paired t test comparisons

mortality (Table 3, $p < 0.10$, Fisher exact test). The only change in our ongoing study of this treatment from that described in the present paper is the insertion of a central venous catheter to facilitate infusion therapy and to allow easy administration of hypertonic glucose if needed to maintain blood sugar levels within the normal range. Hypoglycaemia, the major complication of this therapy, can thus be prevented. The death of one patient, partially related to the insulin infusion, emphasizes the potential for complications with this treatment and the need for careful monitoring of all individuals studied.

Table 7 Blood insulin and glucagon levels (mean ± SD)

	Insulin (µU/ml)		Glucagon (pg/ml)	
	Drug*	Control	Drug†	Control
Baseline	14 ± 8	18 ± 13	338 ± 196	217 ± 132
Week 1	153 ± 126	63 ± 67	1990 ± 642	187 ± 132
Week 2	194 ± 164	71 ± 60	2881 ± 1633	218 ± 124
Week 3	265 ± 146	96 ± 94	3004 ± 2359	291 ± 358

* $p < 0.01$ or greater compared with control during infusion
† $p < 0.005$ or greater compared with control during infusion
(Baker, A. L. et al., 1981. Reprinted, with permission, from Gastroenterology, **80**, 1410)

The improvement in the total serum bilirubin levels and prothrombin times in the insulin and glucagon treated group also suggests that this treatment is beneficial to the liver, despite the absence of significant changes in the other standard liver function tests. Newer tests of discrete liver functions might offer an advantage in monitoring response to therapy with insulin and glucagon. However, the ABT failed to improve significantly in the present study, although it has been shown that this test is useful for assigning a prognosis in alcoholic hepatitis[21]. In the 21 patients who had measurements of amino acid profiles and determination of the branched chain to aromatic amino acid ratios at the beginning and end of the study, no differences could be identified between insulin and glucagon treated and control patients. Likewise, in the small number of patients in whom the alpha fetoprotein levels were studied, values clearly out of the normal range were not found in either group. Although this test may reflect hepatic regeneration in some liver diseases such as hepatitis[15,22], our studies suggest that this test may not be useful for monitoring alcoholic hepatitis patients.

The presumed beneficial effects of insulin and glucagon are probably due to the modifying effects of these hormones on hepatic regeneration, as suggested in recent animal studies[1-5]. However, the precise mechanism of the hepatotrophic effect is unknown[23]. The insulin dose administered in the present study was similar to that utilized in previous animal investigations, but a higher glucagon dose was chosen because of the absence of significant side effects. Higher doses or different schedules of insulin and glucagon administration might conceivably be more beneficial in the treatment of alcoholic hepatitis. Liver biopsies were performed in 5 patients, 3 receiving insulin and glucagon and 2 the control infusion, before and after study. Although histologic evidence of alcoholic hepatitis decreased in all patients, there were no differences between the two groups, perhaps due to the small number of subjects studied. Greater caloric intake might explain the improvement in the insulin and glucagon treated patients. However, the mean daily caloric intake was similar among the 9 insulin and glucagon infused and 7 control patients where accurate calorie counts were recorded.

The results of the present study do not yet justify treatment of alcoholic hepatitis patients with insulin and glucagon. The standard treatment for this disease should continue to be supportive, unless patients can be entered into randomized controlled trials where both the beneficial and harmful effects of this new approach to therapy can be clearly identified.

Acknowledgements

This study was supported in part by a grant from the Novo Research Institute, Copenhagen, Denmark, and by Clinical Research Center Grant RR55-16.

References

1. Marchioro, T. L., Porter, K. A., Dickenson, T. C., Faris, T. D. and Starlz, T. E. (1965). Physiologic requirements for auxiliary liver homotransplantation. *Surg. Gynecol. Obstet.*, **121**, 16
2. Starzl, T. E. (1974). Judd lecture – Portal hepatotrophic factors; a century of controversy. In Najarian, J. S. and Delaney, J. P. (eds.) *Surgery of the Liver, Biliary Tract, and Pancreas*, p. 495 (New York: Intercontinental Medical Book Corp.)
3. Starzl, T. E., Porter, K. A., Watanabe, K. and Putnam, C. W. (1976). Effects of insulin, glucagon, and insulin/glucagon infusions on liver morphology and cell division after complete portacaval shunt in dogs. *Lancet*, **1**, 821
4. Bucher, N. L. R. and Swaffield, M. N. (1975). Regulation of hepatic regeneration in rats by synergistic action of insulin and glucagon. *Proc. Nat. Acad. Sci. U.S.A.*, **72**, 1157
5. Farivar, M., Wands, J. R., Isselbacher, K. J. and Bucher, N. L. R. (1976). Effect of insulin and glucagon on fulminant murine hepatitis. *N. Engl. J. Med.*, **295**, 1517
6. Harinasuta, U., Chomet, B., Ishak, K. and Zimmerman, H. J. (1967). Steatonecrosis–Mallory body type. *Medicine*, **46**, 141
7. Lischner, M. W., Alexander, J. F. and Galambos, J. T. (1971). Natural history of alcoholic hepatitis. I. The acute disease. *Am. J. Dig. Dis.*, **16**, 481
8. Gregory, D. H. and Levi, D. F. (1972). The clinical-pathologic spectrum of alcoholic hepatitis. *Am. J. Dig. Dis.*, **17**, 479
9. Porter, H. P., Simon, F. R., Pope, C. E., Volwiler, W. and Fenster, L. F. (1971). Corticosteroid therapy in severe alcoholic hepatitis: A double-blind drug trial. *N. Engl. J. Med.*, **824**, 1350
10. Morgan, C. R. and Lazarow, A. (1963). Immunoassay of insulin: two antibody system. Plasma insulin levels of normal, subdiabetic, and diabetic rats. *Diabetes*, **12**, 115
11. Kuku, S. F., Jaspan, J. B., Emmanouel, D. S., Zeidler, A., Katz, A. I. and Rubenstein, A. H. (1976). Heterogeneity of plasma glucagon: circulating components in normal subjects and patients with chronic renal failure. *J. Clin. Invest.*, **58**, 742
12. Bircher, J., Kupfer, A., Gikalov, I. and Preisig, R. (1976). Aminopyrine demethylation measured by breath analysis in cirrhosis. *Clin. Pharmacol. Ther.*, **20**, 484

13. Heinrikson, R. L. and Kramer, K. J. (1974). Recent advances in the chemical modification and covalent structural analysis of proteins. In Kniser, E. T. and Kezdy, K. J. (eds.) *Progress in Bioorganic Chemistry*, Vol. 3, pp. 141–250 (New York: John Wiley)

14. Fischer, J. F., Rosen, H. M., Ebeird, A. M., James, J. H., Keane, J. M. and Soeters, P. B. (1977). The effect of normalization of plasma amino acids on hepatic encephalopathy in man. *Surgery*, **80**, 77

15. Bloomer, J. R. (1980). Alpha fetoprotein in nonneoplastic liver diseases. *Dig. Dis. Sci.*, **25**, 241

16. Helman, R. A., Temko, M. H., Nye, S. W. and Fallon H. J. (1971). Alcoholic hepatitis. Natural history and evaluation of prednisone therapy. *Ann. Intern. Med.*, **74**, 311

17. Campra, J. L., Hamlin, E. M., Kirshbaum, R. J., Olivier, M., Redeker, A. G. and Reynolds, T. B. (1973). Prednisone therapy of acute alcoholic hepatitis. Report of a controlled trial. *Ann. Intern. Med.*, **79**, 625

18. Blitzer, B. L., Mutchnick, M. G., Joshi, P. H., Phillips, M. M., Fessel, J. M. and Conn H. O. (1977). Adrenocorticosteroid therapy in alcoholic hepatitis. *Am. J. Dig. Dis.*, **22**, 477

19. Maddrey, W. C., Boitnott, J. K., Bedine, M. S., Weber, F. L., Mezey, E. and White, R. I. (1978). Corticosteroid therapy of alcoholic hepatitis. *Gastroenterology*, **75**, 193

20. Depew, W., Boyer, T., Omata, M., Redeker, A. and Reynolds, T. (1980). Double-blind controlled trial of prednisolone therapy in patients with severe acute alcoholic hepatitis and spontaneous encephalopathy. *Gastroenterology*, **78**, 524

21. Schneider, J. F., Baker, A. L., Haines, N. W., Hatfield, G. and Boyer, J. L. (1980). Aminopyrine N-demethylation: A prognostic test of liver function in patients with alcoholic liver disease. *Gastroenterology*, **79**, 1145

22. Silver, H. K. B., Dencault, J., Gold, P., Thompson, W. G., Shuster, J. and Freedman, S. O. (1974). The detection of α_1-fetoprotein in patients with viral hepatitis. *Cancer Res.*, **34**, 244

23. Sherlock, S. (1976). Portal venous "goodies" and fulminant viral hepatitis. *N. Engl. J. Med.*, **295**, 1535

Address for correspondence

Dr. A. L. Baker,
Director,
Liver Study Unit,
University of Chicago,
950 East 59th Street,
Chicago, IL 60637
USA

DISCUSSION

Hardcastle: For how long did you follow the patients after the study was completed? Was there any difference between the two groups as to the time at which death occurred?

Baker: Our intention, as the study was initially set up, was to follow the patients for six months after the infusions were completed. However, we found a high mortality unrelated to liver disease. One patient burned himself to death when smoking in bed at night, another individual was killed when he ran his car into a bridge abutment, so we really did not think that this analysis was very meaningful, as many deaths were related to alcohol consumption and not to liver disease. If one considers only the deaths which occurred during the three-week study period, when the patients were in the hospital, there was no difference by life table analysis that was any more significant than the overall difference you saw in Table 1.

Okuda: You mentioned the lack of effect on alpha-fetoprotein levels. I have had one patient who I thought responded to insulin and glucagon therapy with a tremendous rise in alpha-fetoprotein. It went as high as 80 000 ng/ml. This was a shocking response, and we thought that this really represented enhanced liver cell regeneration. But this occurred in only one patient. Otherwise we could not demonstrate an increase in alpha-fetoprotein.

Baker: That is interesting. There have been a number of observations suggesting that in chronic hepatitis and in viral hepatitis there may be significant elevations of alpha-fetoprotein, but I am not aware of any published reports of this in fulminant hepatic failure. We were interested in looking at this in this group of patients simply because the possibility existed that insulin and glucagon might stimulate hepatic regeneration and result in increased alpha-fetoprotein levels. A number of studies had previously shown that over a short period of time in the hospital most individuals with alcoholic hepatitis do not respond with an elevation of alpha-fetoprotein, whereas many patients with viral hepatitis and chronic hepatitis do. What these conflicting results in different types of liver disease mean is not completely clear. I am not sure if alpha-fetoprotein really is a marker of regeneration, or if it is an independent phenomenon in the hepatocyte.

Okuda: I think there is pretty good evidence that it does represent regenerative activities of the liver cells, but this applies only to a pathologic state not to a post-hepatectomy condition, and I think only in viral hepatitis, not alcoholic.

Baker: But the absence of elevations in alpha-fetoprotein after partial hepatectomy argues that this protein may not be a marker of hepatic regeneration.

Diamant: Was the glucagon and insulin treatment in your study intermittent or continuous?

Baker: It was continuous for 12 hours a day, beginning in the morning. The patients were not treated at night. Treatment was continued for three weeks.

Diamant: Can the rather large variation you have on the serum levels of glucagon/insulin be explained by the possibility that the dietary regimen was not always kept up? Are the values presented fasting levels in the morning?

167

Baker: The first sample, the baseline one, was a fasting sample. The others represented samples taken with the infusion running, but about four hours after the patient had had breakfast, so that most meal effects should have disappeared.

Diamant: This does not exclude the possibility that large variations might result from the same dose of insulin/glucagon used in different individuals. One should consider monitoring steady state levels by following serum levels, instead of giving a routine dose.

Jaspan: There was in fact quite a lot of variability and I think part of the reason, as Dr. Baker mentioned, is that these patients were receiving glucose infusion and probably, therefore, contributing endogenous insulin. As far as the glucagon is concerned though, the amount given was 200 μg/h; given that the physiologic replacement dose is 4 to 5 μg/h, this is 50 times higher, and, in fact, the plasma values were around 2000 pg/ml, which is 50 times physiologic. So while there was variability due to factors such as pump intermittency and variable hepatic extraction due to variable degrees of liver dysfunction, variable kidney perfusion, and so on, I nevertheless view this as positive rather than negative, since the values were actually reasonably stable given all the other, often greater, variabilities. Insulin levels were much lower and I think the reason for this is that the insulin infusion doses were limited by hypoglycaemia. The levels reached were, in fact, not much greater than would occur after a normal meal in a normal person, and again nutritional status probably had an important influence. In this regard it is noteworthy that the glucagon levels did not change much in the control subjects, while the insulin levels improved quite markedly. This can almost certainly be accounted for by the patient feeling better, eating better, and therefore general nutritional status improving.

Baker: I would emphasize the point that if the patient's arm is bent and the catheter kinks for a period of time, the infusion rate will change. This probably accounts for some of the variability seen. We would certainly like to have seen less variability, but I am not sure that this can be achieved in a patient study.

Bucher: Can you say anything about the nutritional state of the patients? What was their nutritional state when you started your study?

Baker: I am afraid I cannot give you any really systematic data on this point. The dietary intake of the patients at the Clinical Research Center was carefully monitored, and the caloric and protein intake was equal in, I believe, 12 of the insulin and glucagon and 10 of the control patients. However, there was certainly evidence of significant nutritional depletion in the great majority of the patients. Folate deficiency, phosphate deficiency, anaemia and weight loss were very common in the entire group. This might be particularly important in the light of the studies which Dr. Galambos and his group have recently published showing that parenteral nutrition appears to exert a beneficial effect in alcoholic hepatitis.

Bucher: What about endogenous hormone levels before you start treatment? Also, are there any data on effects of nutrition alone, for evaluating changes due to the hormone therapy?

Baker: We do have some data. In the control group there was a slight rise both in insulin and in glucagon levels throughout the three-week duration of the study and part of this effect may well have been nutritional. In the treated group, of course, the levels rose much more dramatically. Essentially there was a doubling of the insulin level and an even steeper increase in the glucagon level.

Miller: Presumably these patients were withdrawn from alcohol during the treatment period. Was there any correlation between improvement and the previous intake of alcohol?

Baker: Let me give you a little more detail about the patients. Some two-thirds of them had a history of taking 100–120 g ethanol per day, that is to say, the equivalent of around twelve cans of beer per day. The other third had a history of consuming large quantities of alcohol for years, without specific quantification. I think it fair to say that all patients in this study probably drank in the region of 100–120 g ethanol per day.

Vilardell: Am I correct in saying that perhaps the sicker the patient the better the chances that this treatment will work?

Baker: That is what our initial data suggest, and that really makes sense, because it is the sickest patient who is at greatest risk of death. If the treatment is going to make any impact on mortality, it is in the patient who has the greatest likelihood of dying that you ought to be able to see the difference.

Jaspan: One should add, however, that in a study such as this, if the patient is too sick he may die even though he receives treatment. Thus applying this treatment to a critically ill and perhaps non-salvageable patient may compromise the ability to demonstrate a true treatment effect in the somewhat less agonal and potentially reversible cases. Also, in this study a treatment death due to hypoglycaemia, which was a side effect of the treatment rather than treatment failure, had an important negative effect on the statistics related to patient deaths.

12

Glucagon and insulin therapy in fulminant hepatic failure in Japan

H. OKA, K. OKITA and K. FUJIWARA

INTRODUCTION

The mortality rate of fulminant hepatitis is extremely high and the therapeutic procedures employed until now have not been satisfactory.

Fulminant hepatitis is a clinical syndrome developing as a result of massive necrosis of the liver cells. Therefore, regeneration of the liver is a principal mechanism for recovery.

Recently, experimental studies[1,2] have demonstrated the synergistic hepatotrophic action of glucagon and insulin, and Baker et al. have reported on a clinical trial in which infusions of glucagon and insulin were used in the treatment of alcoholic hepatitis[3]. These experimental studies and the preliminary findings of Baker et al. led to the suggestion that infusions of glucagon and insulin might be effective in the treatment of fulminant hepatitis.

This therapy has been used clinically for fulminant hepatitis in Japan since 1977. Several authors[4-10] have found it useful, their patients recovering after its use; others have reported unsatisfactory results.

It seems appropriate at this time to make an evaluation of the usefulness of this therapy. Accordingly the records of patients suffering fulminant hepatitis and treated with glucagon and insulin infusions (64 patients) have been collected from eleven medical centres. It is data relating to these 64 cases which are reported here.

ANALYSIS OF THE RECORDS OF 64 CASES OF FULMINANT HEPATITIS TREATED WITH GLUCAGON AND INSULIN

The doses of glucagon and insulin used were generally 1 mg and 10 units respectively. The hormones were dissolved in 500 ml of 5% glucose solution and infused via a peripheral vein for periods of 2–6 h at a time. In more than half of the cases, two or three periods of this treatment were given per day. In some cases different doses of glucagon and/or insulin were used, and in some instances the doses of the hormones were changed following the measurement of blood sugar levels.

In most cases the infusion of glucagon and insulin was started immediately after the onset of hepatic coma or upon admission to hospital. In six cases the infusion was started before the onset of coma when clinical signs and laboratory data, such as a very high serum bilirubin level or an extremely prolonged prothrombin time, suggested the development of severe hepatic dysfunction.

Most of the patients were simultaneously treated with other therapeutic measures. Approximately half were given glucocorticoids and/or fresh-frozen plasma, and in some cases an exchange transfusion, plasmapheresis, or charcoal haemoperfusion was performed.

Of the 64 cases studied, 29 (45.3%) recovered. This survival rate is very high when compared with the rates previously reported in Japan[11] and in other countries. Apparent improvements in hepatic coma were seen in 37.5% of cases, in prothrombin time in 32.8%, and in serum total bilirubin in 25% (Table 1).

Prolongation of prothrombin time is regarded as a good indicator of the increasing severity of hepatic dysfunction. Prothrombin time (%) of 21 cases in the present study was less than 25% when the glucagon and insulin infusions were started; 4 of these 21 cases survived, a survival rate of 19%. In patients whose prothrombin time (%) was higher than 25% when treatment was begun the survival rate was about 60% (Table 2). This result indicates that the glucagon and insulin infusion therapy is not so dramatically effective in patients with extremely severe dysfunction of the liver.

In five cases patients who were recorded as being in grade I coma before therapy was started, and who survived, were evaluated as 'unchanged' in terms of hepatic coma. Serum cholinesterase activity was measured in 45 cases, and an increase observed in 22 (48.9%).

Adverse effects of the glucagon and insulin therapy were: hypokalaemia which occurred in 6 cases, hypoglycaemia 3 cases, nausea 2 cases, and metabolic alkalosis 1 case.

Table 1   Analysis of the records of 64 cases of fulminant hepatitis treated with glucagon and insulin

	No. of patients	%
Hepatic coma		
Improved	24	37.5
Unchanged	17	26.6
Advanced	23	35.9
Prothrombin time		
Improved	21	32.8
Unchanged or prolonged	43	67.2
Serum total bilirubin		
Decreased	16	25.0
Unchanged	26	40.6
Increased	22	34.4
Serum cholinesterase activity		
(recorded in 45 cases)		
Increased	22	48.9
Unchanged	12	26.7
Decreased	11	24.4
Adverse effects		
Hypokalaemia	6	
Hypoglycaemia	3	
Nausea	2	
Metabolic alkalosis	1	

Evaluation of the therapy by the physicians in charge: The therapy proved useful in 25 cases.

Table 2   Prothrombin time (%) when glucagon and insulin therapy was started, and survival rates

	< 25 %	25–40 %	> 40 %
Number of cases	21	21	12
Number of surviving	4	13	7
Survival rate (%)	19.0	61.9	58.3

The therapy was evaluated by the physicians in charge as having been useful in 25 cases.

The survival rate in these patients treated with glucagon and insulin, 45.3 %, is considerably higher than that of 16.5 % found by Takahashi et al.[11] in a nation-wide survey of fulminant hepatitis in Japan in the period 1974–76, i.e., before glucagon and insulin therapy began to be used in this connection.

The prognosis of fulminant hepatitis is known to be affected by age, aetiology, and degree of hepatic dysfunction and coma. In addition, Takahashi et al.[11] found the prognosis to be better in the acute form of the disease, i.e., when coma develops within 10 days of onset, than in the subacute form when it develops later. The data of the two studies were therefore analysed to see if the difference in the survival rates could be explained by any of these factors.

The age distribution of the patients in the two studies is shown in Figure 1. The distribution patterns are not dissimilar. In the national survey the survival

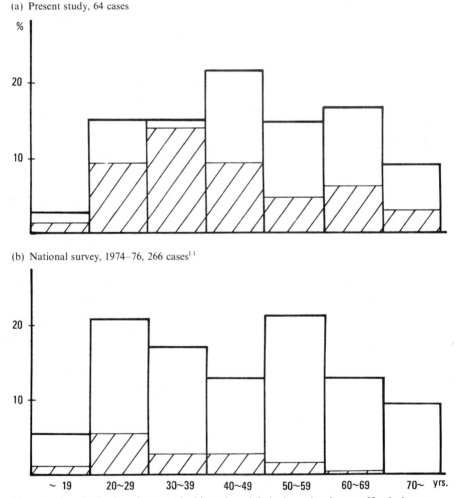

(a) Present study, 64 cases

(b) National survey, 1974–76, 266 cases[11]

Figure 1 Age distribution of cases (a) in this study and (b) in the national survey. Hatched areas indicate percentage of each age group surviving

rate of older patients was extremely low; only 1 of the 66 patients aged 60 or more survived. In patients treated with glucagon and insulin the survival rate in the older age groups was very much higher.

As far as aetiological factors are concerned, higher survival rates are usually observed in patients with fulminant hepatitis induced by halothane or other drugs, while the prognosis of fulminant viral hepatitis is generally extremely poor. In both aetiological groups the survival rates of patients in the present study were much higher than those in the national survey, indicating that the difference in survival rates of the two studies is not due to differences in the aetiology of the disease.

Distribution of the grades of hepatic coma when treatment was started and the survival rate of each group are shown in Table 3. In the national survey the survival rate was very poor in patients with grade IV coma; it was much higher in the grade IV coma patients treated with glucagon and insulin. Approximately 4/6 of patients with grades I or II coma recovered with glucagon and insulin treatment, compared to 1/6 of patients with the same grade of coma in the national survey. In 6 cases in the present study treatment with glucagon and insulin was started before the onset of hepatic coma, severe liver dysfunction having been diagnosed from laboratory and clinical tests; only 1 of these 6 patients survived.

In the national survey survival rates of the acute form and of the subacute form of fulminant hepatitis were 22.3% and 9.4% respectively. In the present study 33 cases were of the acute form and 31 the subacute form; the survival rates were 51.5% and 38.7% respectively. The described glucagon and insulin infusion therapy was effective in both forms of the disease.

As the prognosis of fulminant hepatitis is extremely poor, several therapeutic procedures are usually used simultaneously. In the present study glucocorticoids, exchange transfusion, charcoal haemoperfusion, and other

Table 3 Grades of hepatic coma when therapy was started, and survival rates

	0	I	II	III	IV
(a) Present study					
Number of patients	6 (1)	7 (5)	15 (10)	17 (4)	19 (9)
Survival rate (%)	16.7	71.4	66.7	23.5	47.4
(b) National survey					
Number of patients	5 (1)	41 (5)	69 (13)	72 (18)	79 (6)
Survival rate (%)	20.0	12.2	18.8	25.0	7.6

No. surviving in parentheses

measures were used in conjunction with the glucagon and insulin therapy. As a result it is difficult to evaluate the usefulness of individual therapies. An evaluation of the described glucagon and insulin therapy is to some extent possible, however, if one compares the survival rates of patients treated with certain therapies in the national survey with those of patients treated with the same therapies plus glucagon and insulin in the present study. The survival rate of patients treated with glucocorticoids alone was 14.4%; in contrast, that of patients treated with glucocorticoids plus glucagon and insulin was 60% (Table 4). In the cases of exchange transfusion + glucocorticoids, and of charcoal haemoperfusion, the addition of therapy with glucagon and insulin did not so markedly improve the prognosis; slightly higher survival rates were nevertheless observed (Table 4).

MULTI-CENTRE DOUBLE-BLIND CONTROLLED TRIAL OF GLUCAGON AND INSULIN THERAPY

The above findings clearly indicate the usefulness of glucagon and insulin therapy in cases of fulminant hepatitis. The importance of proving the value of therapies by conducting controlled studies is appreciated. For this reason we are currently conducting a multi-centre double-blind controlled trial of this therapy in connection with hepatitis. The study is being conducted in patients with a severe type of acute hepatitis, not fulminant hepatitis since for us the

Table 4   Therapeutic measures used, and survival rates

Therapeutic measures used	No. of cases	No. surviving	Survival rate (%)
Glucocorticoids (National survey)	125	18	14.4
Glucocorticoids + glucagon and insulin (Present study)	25	15	60.0
Exchange transfusion + glucocorticoids (National survey)	31	7	22.6
Exchange transfusion + glucocorticoids + glucagon and insulin (Present study)	6	2	33.3
Charcoal haemoperfusion (National survey)	19	5	26.3
Charcoal haemoperfusion + glucagon and insulin (Present study)	10	3	30.0

conducting of such a trial in patients with this disease would hardly be acceptable from an ethical point of view. The patients chosen for the study are those with acute hepatitis, with a prothrombin time (%) between 30% and 60%, and a maximum of grade III hepatic coma. Patients with severe complications, such as malignancies, severe infection, gastrointestinal bleedings or disseminated intravascular coagulation, and those over 70 years of age are excluded, as are patients being treated with glucocorticoids, heparin, fresh plasma, amino acid infusion, exchange transfusion, or charcoal haemoperfusion. Patients fulfilling the study criteria after informed consent to enter the study are randomly assigned to the glugacon and insulin group or to the control group. The doses of glucagon and insulin are 1 mg and 10 units respectively; the two hormones are dissolved in 500 ml of 5% glucose and infused twice per day for one week. The parameters being measured are listed in Table 5. The study began in July 1981 and is still in progress.

Table 5   Parameters being measured before, during and after the study (* before and after only)

---

*1) Blood count: RBC, WBC, platelet, Hb, Ht

2) Blood chemistry:
   Total protein, albumin, bilirubin (total and direct),
   cholesterol, alkaline phosphatase,
   cholinesterase, GOT, GPT,
   α-fetoprotein, blood sugar, urea-N,
   PO_4^-, Na^+, K^+, Cl^-,
   α-HS-glycoprotein, pre-albumin

3) Prothrombin time
   (hepaplastin test or thrombotest)

4) Histological examination, when possible

5) Adverse effects

References

1. Bucher, N. L. R. and Swaffield, M. N. (1975). Regulation of hepatic regeneration in rats by synergistic action of insulin and glucagon. *Proc. Natl. Acad. Sci. USA*, **72**, 1157
2. Bucher, N. L. R. (1976). Insulin, glucagon, and the liver. *Adv. Enzyme Regul.*, **15**, 221
3. Baker, A. L., Jaspan, J. B., Haines, N. W., Hatfield, G. E., Krager, P. S., Schneider, J. F. and the University of Chicago Medical House staff (1981). A randomized clinical trial of insulin and glucagon infusion for treatment of alcoholic hepatitis: Progress report in 50 patients. *Gastroenterology*, **80**, 1410
4. Okita, K., Matsuda, S., Hata, K., Morimoto, T., Sasaki, M., Fukumoto, Y., Kodama, T. and Takemoto, T. (1979). Clinical use of glucagon and insulin in therapy of fulminant hepatic failure. *Gastroenterol. Jpn.*, **14**, 453

5. Tanaka, N., Noda, Y., Hirai, N., Ikeda, T., Okai, T., Nakagawa, H., Iwata, A., Unoura, M., Kumagai, M., Morita, N., Kameda, S., Nishimura, K., Kato, Y., Kobayashi, K. and Hattori, N. (1980). Insulin-glucagon therapy on acute hepatitis. *Acta Hepatol. Jpn.*, **28**, 1626
6. Okita, K., Aibe, T., Kaya, S., Miyazaki, M., Yamaguchi, M., Fujii, R., Noda, K., Fuji, T., Fukumoto, Y., Kodama, T., Takemoto, T., Oka, T. and Makisaka, Y. (1978). A study on the interaction of the therapeutic agents for hepatitis to the damaged liver cells. 3: Application of glucagon-insulin therapy to the treatment of acute and chronic hepatic failure. *Acta Hepatol. Jpn.*, **19**, 854
7. Matsuda, S. (1980). Studies on glucagon-insulin therapy for the treatment of acute liver failure. 1: Clinical studies. *Acta Hepatol. Jpn.*, **21**, 730
8. Hosokawa, Y., Suga, M., Yokoyama, Y., Kinoshita, H., Anzai, T., Fujisawa, Y., Fujishima, A., Fujita, H. and Saito, M. (1980). A case of fulminant hepatitis cured with the glucagon-insulin treatment. *Acta Hepatol. Jpn.*, **21**, 1352
9. Watanabe, A., Higashi, T., Hayashi, S., Obata, T., Endo, H., Nagashima, H., Morimoto, C. and Suzuki, S. (1980). A survived case of fulminant hepatitis with a trial of simultaneous infusions of insulin and glucagon. *Acta Hepatol. Jpn.*, **21**, 1044
10. Suga, M., Hosokawa, Y., Yokoyama, Y., Kinoshita, H., Anzai, T., Fujishima, A., Fujita, H., Saito, M. and Shirai, Y. (1980). Treatment of hepatic insufficiency with glucagon-insulin. Part 1: Improvement of hepatic encephalopathy and changes of blood ammonia levels by glucagon-insulin treatment. *Acta Hepatol. Jpn.*, **21**, 1631
11. Takahashi, Y., Shimizu, M. and Kosaka, M. (1979). Nationwide statistics of severe hepatitis (fulminant hepatitis). (In Japanese) *Saishin Igaku*, **34**, 2285

Address for correspondence

Dr H. Oka,
First Department of Internal Medicine,
Faculty of Medicine, University of Tokyo,
3-1 Hongo 7-chome,
Bunkyo-ku,
Tokyo 113, Japan

DISCUSSION

Baker: I have a question regarding the criteria for inclusion in your controlled trial. I noticed that you excluded patients who had received plasma. Yet, I take it you are not excluding patients who received blood. Is that right?

Oka: No. All patients receiving plasma or blood are excluded.

Baker: What is your reason for that?

Oka: One of the parameters in our study is prothrombin time. If plasma is given to the patient, the prothrombin time will be altered. I think the volume of plasma very important. For this reason all patients who had exchange plasma transfusion are excluded.

Baker: I certainly think it wise to exclude patients who have had exchange transfusion. My only concern is that by excluding all patients who have had plasma or blood transfusion your patient population will be unduly limited.

Skucas: Can you explain why you chose the dose of 1 mg glucagon and 10 units insulin?

Oka: There is no reason other than the fact that this dose – 1 mg glucagon and 10 units insulin twice per day – had been satisfactorily used in Japan in the past. Dr. Baker was using a similar dose, 2.4 mg glucagon and 24 units insulin per 24 hours, which is the same ratio that we have used. Note that this is the dose per treatment, and that we treat twice per day, once in the morning and once in the evening. The dose per day is 2 mg glucagon and 20 units insulin.

Miller: The matter of the ideal dose is an unresolved one. I do not know if anyone has done this, but perhaps if one was to take an animal, give it an LD_{50} dose of carbon tetrachloride, or something of that nature, and then titrate out a dose at different levels, it might be possible to arrive at some conclusions as to an appropriate dose. I do not disagree with what you have done, it is just that I think the doses that many of us are using are not very soundly based.

Jaspan: The problem with doing that is two-fold. One is metabolic clearance, that in animals differs very much. Secondly, in humans one is often limited by hypoglycaemia, although this would not be as much of a concern in animals. The point is well taken: we do not know what the optimal doses are. I do not know, however, how best to establish them, for, as we have already seen today, it is difficult to find an appropriate animal model.

Bucher: We always gave glucose along with the insulin when high doses were employed, to prevent death from hypoglycemia (Bucher, N. L. R., *et al.* (1978). In Ciba Foundation Symposium 55 *Hepatotrophic Factors*, pp. 95–109. New York: Elsevier, Excerpta Medica, North Holland.

Jaspan: The trouble is that one gets into problems with thrombophlebitis when one is using hypertonic glucose.

Bucher: That is true.

Baker: That is one improvement we made in our study, which I mentioned before. We now insert a central line for our studies, which makes it much easier to give the hormones and to give the appropriate amount of glucose. Our initial insulin dose was based on Starzl's studies in dogs (Starzl, T. E. *et al.* (1975). *Lancet*, **2**, 1241 and (1976). *Lancet*, **1**, 821), on a weight basis. I do not think anyone knows what the right dose is in man, but I do not know how to determine the right dose in an animal model either.

Bucher: But Starzl never got an effect with glucagon. His experiments were all in dogs which react more slowly than rats to liver deficits, and also the experimental conditions were different from ours. Our cell culture studies suggest that the metabolic state of the cells may be an important determinant on the effects of glucagon on hepatic DNA synthesis.

Baker: I should like to ask Dr. Oka about the rationale for the administration of two cycles of treatment per day in his controlled trial. I believe that each cycle lasts for 4 hours. Is that right?

Oka: The first cycle of treatment is in the morning, the second in the afternoon, and each one lasts 2 to 4 hours.

Baker: I should like to ask you also your rationale.

Oka: We really had no valid reason other than the fact that in our retrospective report there were 64 cases treated that way, so for the prospective controlled study we decided to follow a similar pattern.

General discussion

A. ORIOL BOSCH and F. VILARDELL

Oriol Bosch: I should like to suggest that in this general discussion session we try to cover three main topics: physiopharmacology, motility, and liver regeneration. Let us begin with physiopharmacology, where the basic questions, it seems to me, concern circulating plasma levels, dosages, the bioavailability of glucagon, the analogues, and, what I consider to be a particularly important matter, that of the glucagon receptors. Let us take the receptors first. I would like to ask what is known about glucagon receptors and how these are modulated. This question, if I have to justify it, is asked because, at least in endocrinology, the down regulation mechanism of hormones through the exhaustion of receptors is something we have been learning a lot about in the last few years. It seems that by using the wrong dosage or the wrong schedule one can obtain counter-results to the ones one is trying to achieve; this is because one exhausts the receptors and does not give sufficient time for their regeneration or replacement. I should like to know if any information is available on glucagon receptors in this respect.

Jaspan: Well, the data that there is, and there is not very much, has mainly come from two laboratories, those of Recant and Bhathena and of Felig and Soman. Felig and Soman showed that physiologic hyperglucagonaemia can down regulate the glucagon receptor quite markedly (Soman, V. and Felig, P. (1978). *J. Clin. Invest.*, **61**, 552). Both groups did their studies in streptozotocin diabetic rats, but whereas Recant and Bhathena used the whole hepatocyte (Bhathena, S. I. *et al.* (1978). *J. Clin. Invest.*, **61**, 1488), Felig and Soman used liver membranes, and in fact the two groups found diametrically opposite results – in one study the receptors went up and in the other they went down. Unfortunately, some of the work which has been done in this field is open to criticism, and perhaps the only thing one can really say at the moment is that this whole matter is one which warrants further investigation. It is a subject which we, in Chicago,

181

would very much like to study. We would like to know what relation the receptor has to degradation, and what happens in situations of stress, exercise, feeding, fasting, protein-rich meals, and so on. At the moment it seems that very little is known.

Diamant: I think one is probably talking about two different things when one speaks about receptors for the metabolic effects of glucagon and receptors for the spasmolytic action. I do not think that anyone knows exactly where the receptors for the spasmolytic action are located, how they look, or how they bind. It would be very interesting to make an histological examination with immunoassays to see, in the gut wall for example, to which structures glucagon does actually bind. To my knowledge, no-one has yet done this. To go back to the original question, several groups have shown that in the plasma membrane cyclic GMP dissociates glucagon from its receptor (Birnbaumer, L. and Pohl, S. L. (1973). *J. Biol. Chem.*, **248**, 2056). There is, therefore, an interaction between cyclic GMP and glucagon in relation to the binding. I do not think, however, that this has anything to do with the up or down regulation of the receptors. Whether or not cyclic GMP might also influence the binding of glucagon-(1-21)-peptide and thus reverse its spasmolytic action is not known.

Jaspan: I think that one should mention also that it may turn out that the pharmacologic actions of glucagon are not receptor-mediated at all, and that they do not depend upon cyclic AMP. It could be that the action is a direct one. This is an important matter; one which really should be looked into.

Oriol Bosch: What about the question of the bioavailability of glucagon or of glucagon analogues? We have heard about a few of these analogues. Professor Diamant has worked with the 1-21 fraction. What does the future hold in this respect?

Diamant: That is a question which I should like to ask to the clinicians present. Is there a need for a fragment with a specific spasmolytic effect, a fragment with no metabolic effects?

Hardcastle: What I think is needed for therapeutic purposes is a form which we could give either subcutaneously or intramuscularly, which would be a long-acting depot glucagon. I think this would be a great advance. Is there any likelihood of such a preparation becoming available in the near future, either of glucagon itself or of a fragment?

Diamant: Zinc protamine glucagon is available already, but frankly it has not had the dramatic extension of duration of effects that one had hoped for. At the present time we are looking at various new immobilization procedures which would allow the slow release of glucagon at a constant velocity. There is obviously a need for such a preparation, for out-patients for instance. It is something which is, so to say, on the drawing board.

Skucas: As far as radiology is concerned, we have been able to give glucagon intramuscularly for a number of years now. I think Professor Miller has shown that an intramuscular injection of approximately 2 mg is essentially equivalent to one of 0.25–0.5 mg given intravenously as far as the intensity of action is concerned, but that the intravenous dose does not last as long. Some radiological examinations take a considerable amount of time, and in these instances an intramuscular dose is ideal. The reason that most of us have now switched to the intravenous route is one of cost. It is prohibitively expensive to routinely give, say, 2 mg glucagon i.m. to all patients.

Miller: I agree with Dr. Skucas. I also agree with Professor Hardcastle; I can see real advantages from the therapeutic point of view in the availability of a long-acting depot glucagon. What I personally would like to see, however – and this is not a difference of opinion, but a wish for a preparation for a different purpose, diagnostic as opposed to therapeutic – is something along the lines of the glucagon-(1-21)-peptide. I would like to see something which does not act on certain organs (the kidney, for instance), which is short-acting and can be titrated to a very small degree, and which will relax the gastrointestinal tract, but leave the rest of the body alone. I would certainly like to work with something like the glucagon-(1-21)-peptide.

Diamant: Work on the glucagon-(1-21)-peptide is quite far advanced. It could probably be used in man now, at least for acute administration. When I asked about the need for glucagon preparations to do specific jobs, however, I was really thinking more about subjects such as those described by Dr. Daniel, those with colonic disease, for instance, when one would like a treatment which would last for 2–3 days. A preparation specifically devised for that purpose could be very useful, I would think.

Rey: We do, of course, need both types of preparation. In radiology and endoscopy we need to inject intravenously for a short-acting effect. Intramuscular injection is not always suitable – not in ERCP for instance. In some clinical situations, however, certainly in some of those about which Dr. Daniel spoke, or when treating patients with biliary pain or suspected benign Oddi stenosis, a longer-acting glucagon would indeed be useful, but one without metabolic effects.

Vilardell: In your field, Dr. Rey, could you envisage introducing a catheter into the common bile duct, and using, let us say, a slow release of intramuscular glucagon, leaving it there for 24 h in order to see the variations in common bile duct pressure over that period? Do you think this would be possible?

Rey: It is highly possible. Cotton, in London, has used this technique a lot. He places a transnasal biliary catheter in patients with cholangitis, just after performing an endoscopic sphincterotomy (Cotton, P. B. *et al.* (1979). *Gut*, **20**, 285). It must, therefore, be quite possible to introduce a catheter into the common bile duct, to withdraw the duodenoscope, and to give whatever substances one wishes for 2 or 3 days.

Vilardell: And to take pressures?

Rey: Yes, to take pressures too. But with this kind of system we are able to record only the pressure in front of the side-holed end, so, as the catheter would stay in the common bile duct, we would be able to record only biliary pressure.

Baker: I should like to mention another possible use for a glucagon analogue, and that is in connection with the broad group of cholestatic liver diseases. Individually these diseases are, I suppose, fairly rare, but the pathogenesis often extends over a prolonged period of months or even years. It seems to me that a drug which stimulates bile flow might well be effective in ameliorating or reversing some aspects of these diseases. I am talking about disorders like sclerosing cholangitis, frequently seen in inflammatory bowel disease, primary biliary cirrhosis, and cystic fibrosis, where there are often, not true cholesterol stones in the sense of retained common duct stones, but concretions or ill-defined stones. If these could be flushed out over a period of time it might well be to the benefit of patients. We do not yet have a really effective treatment for this. Phenobarbital and cholesteramine are used at present; they are helpful to some extent, but not ideal.

Diamant: Maybe somebody could give me an opinion as to whether or not we are limited by the dosages of glucagon which we can prescribe today, meaning that if we had a glucagon fragment which did not have metabolic effects we could give much higher doses which might result in improved effects. I know that Professor Miller has shown that in the gut the maximal spasmolytic action is obtained with 0.1 mg, but is the situation the same, I wonder, in the biliary tract? Do you not think it possible that one could induce an enhanced gall bile flow together with enhanced relaxation by increasing the dose to levels we do not use today?

Miller: It is possible, but we shall always need two forms of glucagon preparations, a short-acting one for diagnostic purposes and short-term therapy, and a longer-acting one for long-term therapy.

Diamant: I was thinking more of the glucagon-(1-21)-peptide, which might be given in dosages of, say, 25 or 50 mg. I wonder how you would view that prospect.

Hardcastle: I think one has first got to know a good deal more about what happens when one gives these big doses of glucagon. For instance, I showed you some data on the migrating motor complex; it is a very interesting observation, but we do not really know *why* this happens. It may well be that many other gut hormones change when one throws this sort of big pharmacological spanner into the works. I am not sure that very big doses are necessarily a good thing. I am not sure, incidentally, that we should carry on with the double-blind studies we are doing at the moment in biliary colic and so on, using high doses. I think there is much to be said for treating, say, one hundred cases, and then, when a good effect is seen, treating the next hundred with a lower dose. I wonder what the rest of you feel about this.

Jaspan: It would certainly make good sense to do dose–response curves at the pilot study stage, because there may well be a maximum dose above which one does not need to go, and perhaps should not.

Daniel: When I began using glucagon in colonic disorders some ten years or so ago, I made observations on the effect of bolus injections on intracolonic pressure. My recollection is that an injection is followed very quickly by a fall in pressure, but that this fall is transient. What I should like to know is how long can the spasmolytic effect of glucagon be maintained? I ask this question because I am wondering if glucagon would be helpful after sutured colonic anastomosis. In that situation one would need to be sure that the effect was very long-acting. Does the effect exhaust itself, or does the body produce a barrier to further injections, or what?

Jaspan: Well, metabolically, there have been data to show that in the face of continued hyperglucagonaemia, glucose output by the liver does become refractory. I think that in the pharmacological sphere one may have to be specific in terms of delimiting the duration of the spasmolytic action. I think that the transient effect which you saw may have been due to the fact that a peak was rapidly reached and then rapidly abated. It would be interesting to know what would happen in this situation if one gave a bolus followed by infusion.

Hardcastle: Perhaps I can partly answer that, at least as far as our model is concerned, the dog ureter. One can certainly produce cessation of peristalsis with the initial bolus, but it is not possible to maintain this for long with intravenous infusions, however high the dose. Very high doses do delay the return of peristalsis, but only for a rather short period of time. I would say that 20 minutes' respite would be about the maximum one could achieve. As far as the dog ureter is concerned, one cannot block peristalsis indefinitely.

Baker: I think there is a lot of heterogeneity in the response of various organs. We have conducted studies in the dog in which we infused glucagon and measured the response of bile secretion over a 4 h period. We gave a dose of 200 µg/kg body weight, and we found that, although there was a slight exhaustion over the 4 h observation period, the bile secretion rate was pretty well maintained throughout. This is a pharmacologic dose, but it does suggest that the effect of glucagon, at least on bile flow, could be sustained for a considerable period of time.

Jaspan: We found a similar thing in portal blood flow in the dog. Initially the flow went up, of course. Subsequently, with the continuous infusion of glucagon, it settled at a level about half-way between base line and peak.

Daniel: Over what period of time was that, Dr Jaspan?

Jaspan: Over 15–30 minutes.

Christiansen: I would just add to this discussion that the acid inhibition by intravenous infusion of glucagon appears to continue as long as the infusion continues. We have infused glucagon for about 4 h and seen a steady inhibition over that period.

Vilardell: What about glucagon 'snuff'? Has anyone tried that?

Diamant: It is certainly an attractive idea. Some interesting work is being done on this route of administration with certain other peptides: LH-RH as a contraceptive, for example, CCK-8 for pancreatitis, and so on. We have done a few studies with glucagon and the various fragments in animals, but our work is at a very preliminary stage, and I have no information as to how efficiently the glucagon passes over to the blood. It does, however, remain an interesting thought.

Miller: What about implantable pumps, such as there are for insulin? Could such a pump be developed for glucagon?

Diamant: I am not sure that the insulin pumps have yet been proven superior to multi-injections; some investigators have found them of no special benefit. One can, nevertheless, see that pumps might have a future for chronic diseases such as diabetes. I doubt, however, that one would like to use an implantable pump when one wants to treat a patient for just a few days, as is usually the case, at least at the present time, for glucagon.

Christiansen: May I ask what is perhaps a naïve question? Is it really impossible today to manufacture glucagon or glucagon analogues for administration by the peroral route?

Diamant: That is certainly not a naïve question, because in many ways that would be the optimal route of administration. It does seem, however, that it is not possible without doing a great deal of ingenious substitution work on the molecule, as in the present form the molecule would be broken down by the proteolytic enzymes. For the present, one has to forget that route, I am afraid, and think of other possibilities.

Jaspan: We have spoken today about 'physiologic', 'pharmacologic' and 'super-pharmacologic' levels of glucagon. I should like, if I may, to turn the discussion towards a consideration of the levels about which we are really talking, and to thoughts as to how one should monitor the responses to the doses being given. Perhaps I could start off with the physiologic level. The normal physiologic range is 50–150 pg/ml, i.e. 15–45 picomolar. Let us take 100 pg/ml, or 30 picomolar, as being the middle of the physiologic range. A maximally stimulated physiologic level, such as after Dr. Christiansen's protein meal, or after exercise, or following myocardial infarction, though that must border on pathologic stress, is around 250–500 pg/ml, or 75–150 picomolar, an increase of 5 to 10 times. Physiologic replacement doses (for example following pancreatectomy in a patient, replacement therapy to attain the normal 100 pg/ml level) is usually 1 ng/kg a minute, or, in a 75 kg man, 4–5 µg an hour. Dr. Baker and I, in our study, gave 200 µg an hour, or 2.4 mg over 12 hours, which is some 40–50 times higher. It is important, because of heterogeneity considerations, to be sure that what one has infused is the physiologic hormone, because it can bind to protein, be degraded, and so on. In our study, during infusion in certain patients, we measured glucagon profiles and found, reassuringly, that 95+ % of the glucagon present in the circulation was identical to the infused compound, and that it had not undergone significant biologic transformation. I think that after a bolus dose of 1 mg glucagon – and this again will depend very much on how rapidly the injection is given and on the metabolic status of the animal or human – the levels would reach peaks of about 10 000 to 25 000 pg/ml. When, therefore, like Professor Miller, one gives 0.1 mg, I think that one will quickly reach a peak of 2 to 3000 pg/ml; this will rapidly decline, because of the half-life of about 4 minutes, and physiologic levels will probably be reached within 30 minutes.

Skucas: The effect of glucagon, and its half-life, are probably not the same in the gut as in other organ systems. When you mentioned 30 minutes were you referring to the gut?

Jaspan: I was, in fact, referring to plasma. If one looks at portal blood flow in the dog, when one injects a bolus of glucagon while measuring portal flow with electro-magnetic flow probes, one sees that the flow quickly increases. After the bolus injection, it goes down fairly rapidly. When one continues the administration of glucagon via an infusion, the level does not stay at its peak, but settles after some 15–30 minutes at a level approximately half-way between the base line and the peak, as I mentioned earlier. I think you are correct in saying that the biologic half-life, as measured in the plasma, probably does not correlate with physiologic or pharmacologic actions; this is because the hormone binds or has an action which is generated even though it has disappeared

186

from the plasma. It is a difficult thing to quantitate mathematically or measure biologically.

Skucas: It is extremely difficult and very complex, because even in different parts of the gut there are different actions, and different doses of glucagon are required to achieve the same effect. The action of glucagon on the gut and, say, hyperglycaemia levels, do not really correspond either; there is a great deal of variation.

Jaspan: I agree with that. There are also species differences, as we have heard, and many other complicating factors. I am afraid that at the present time one can do little more than make intelligent guesses.

Hardcastle: Changing the subject somewhat, I would like to know what degree of insulin contamination there is in the glucagon we use.

Jaspan: We have checked this routinely by immunoassay and found no insulin at all.

Hardcastle: I asked this question because if the glucagon did contain any insulin, theoretically these doses could immunize the patient to insulin, which would lead to problems should the patient later become diabetic and need insulin.

Vilardell: Let us now move on a little, away from the physiology and pharmacodynamics of glucagon, to clinical matters. We have already mentioned several fields in which glucagon might be of use. Let us now discuss this matter further. Let us do so by taking the gastrointestinal tract in a sequential fashion, starting perhaps with the esophagus. Are there any conditions in the esophagus in which glucagon could be of use? Unfortunately, it does not seem to be of any help for esophageal diffuse spasm, because, as we have heard today, it does not seem to affect the muscle of the body of the esophagus. This is a pity, for although diffuse spasm is not a common disease, it is a disturbing one, and one which is very difficult to treat. There is no successful medical treatment available for it at present, and the surgeons with their myotomies, although they have been quite successful with achalasia, have not been very successful with diffuse spasm. Is there, I wonder, anything happening in the esophagus for which we think that glucagon may be helpful?

Miller: As I understand it, there are no polypeptide receptors in the body of the esophagus. This is almost certainly one of the reasons why one does not see an effect there.

Diamant: Yes, that is probably right.

Vilardell: What about the lower esophageal sphincter?

Miller: Glucagon certainly has an effect on the sphincter; its use in treating food impaction is evidence of this. Some people, I understand, have also found it to bring relief in cases of achalasia. I have also heard of it being used when trying to distinguish between carcinoma of the stomach involving the esophagus, and carcinoma basically of the esophagus but involving the stomach, the theory being, I believe, that if the lower esophageal sphincter can be relaxed with glucagon, the carcinoma must be in the stomach rather than in the esophagus. I understand, however, that there is only a very little data on this, by no means enough to be conclusive.

Rey: Do you think, Professor Miller, that glucagon would be useful in connection with the endoscopic treatment of achalasia? We now treat this condition by endoscopic dilatation. I wonder if you think that glucagon would be helpful after that.

Miller: Yes, I do. As a matter of fact I know of a case of perforation of the esophagus during endoscopy which could almost certainly have been avoided had glucagon been used.

Hardcastle: I am not quite sure what you mean, Dr. Rey. Are you thinking of using glucagon at the time of dilatation or afterwards? Professor Miller implied that it could be helpful during the procedure. How do you think it might be of help later?

Rey: Quite often, although the dilatation procedure itself has been successful, one sees a recurrence of the stenosis after, say 3 or 6 months, or perhaps a year, and one is then obliged to repeat the procedure.

Vilardell: On the subject of achalasia, however, it seems to me that some 15–20% of patients do not do well whatever one tries. I wonder if, by using something like glucagon, one could not identify these patients in advance. If, for instance, one found no response to glucagon, one would know that there was little point in attempting dilatation. Perhaps it could also be that when there is a response this could help one in treating the patient, especially if one uses a graded instrument when performing dilatation. One could then dilate progressively, and perform several dilatations in a row, say four or five in the course of a week. This is what Vantrappen in Belgium does, with extremely good results.

Hardcastle: Do we in fact know exactly what the effect of glucagon is on the sphincter in achalasia? We are talking about it being 'useful' but do we know exactly what effect it has?

Vilardell: Maybe that is something we do indeed need to establish. This is the purpose of a discussion such as this – to identify situations in which glucagon might be of help, and to establish what things we still need to know about it.

Diamant: Do you think that a controlled clinical trial would be useful if it helped to establish this point?

Vilardell: Most probably, yes.

Diamant: What about food impaction due to esophagitis? It is known that glucagon can be helpful in this connection. We should perhaps just mention this whilst we are talking about the esophagus.

Miller: Yes. There have been several reports on this subject. The treatment is not successful in all cases, not by any means, but it is certainly worth trying. I would prefer glucagon to some of the other preparations which are sometimes used today. It often helps to avoid endoscopy too, which is another reason to try it. I believe it is successful in something like 50% of cases.

Rey: Professor Miller, as a radiologist, tries to avoid endoscopy, of course, but I am an endoscopist. I feel that when there is an impaction of food the patient has almost

188

certainly got some abnormality in the esophagus: a carcinoma, esophagitis, or something else. In my opinion one has to do two things: first, one has to remove the food impaction, but then one is obliged to see what has happened in the esophagus to cause that problem. One needs to perform an endoscopy in any case.

Miller: I do not disagree with you, Dr Rey, but I do think there is much to be said for doing the endoscopy later, in much safer conditions. First, maybe with a little barium, have a good look, get the food passed into the stomach, and then, under more ideal conditions, examine the patient further. I think this also applies – jumping ahead a little – to the stomach, the duodenum, and the colon.

Skucas: Just a brief comment on endoscopy and food impaction. I think I can count on my fingers the number of cancers which have been missed by endoscopy – there have been very few – but the matter can be complicated when the endoscopist is asked to report on the cause of the problem at the same time as he is trying to deal with the food impaction, because a tumour can in fact be hidden by the bolus of food. I agree with Professor Miller. The primary thing is to remove the bolus and then, at leisure, in a day or a week, one can perform a definitive examination. In my opinion the two functions should be completely separated.

Rey: This is what we do.

Baker: I was impressed by the slides which Professor Miller showed this morning illustrating the way in which these boluses can be made to pass. I wonder, Professor Diamant, if there is not some way, short of a clinical study, in which this could be made into a reasonable indication for glucagon, perhaps by the collection of information in a systematic way. In my opinion it is extremely difficult to do controlled trials on a problem like this. I think, to sound a note of caution, that complications can easily arise. I would, for example, be rather frightened to do what I have heard of some people doing, of trying to get the bolus to come out by using glucagon to induce vomiting. I really think that is something which should be discouraged.

Vilardell: There is a condition in the elderly, sometimes brought about by people, particularly women, taking too much bulk laxatives (mucilloids), which some clinicians have come to term 'presby-esophagus', a condition of the esophagus in old age. I do not know if glucagon would be of any help in this connection.

Rey: Has anyone any experience of using glucagon in children? Children are somewhat prone to swallowing odd things, and these do sometimes get stuck in the esophagus. It would be nice if by using glucagon one could avoid endoscopy and general anaesthesia in such cases.

Miller: There have been some reports of glucagon being used for this; cases in which, after glucagon, the coin or whatever moved into the stomach and was then passed normally. I am not saying that this is the best method of treatment, but as an emergency measure, in the middle of the night say, it would not necessarily be a bad thing to try.

Vilardell: Let us now proceed further down the gastrointestinal tract, to the stomach. Dr. Christiansen has shown that glucagon has an anti-secretory effect here. What does this mean in clinical terms? Do you, for instance, see a role for glucagon in the treatment of peptic ulcer?

Christiansen: Well, until it is possible to manufacture a form which can be taken by the peroral route, I do not think that glucagon will have any great value in this field. It is possible that it could be of help in cases of acute bleeding ulcer. There have been a few controlled studies which have shown cimetidine to have negative effect on bleeding ulcers, one must say that. This does not necessarily mean that glucagon would have a good effect; we do not know what its mechanism of action is. It would, however, certainly be an attractive drug to study for this purpose.

Hardcastle: Do we know the effect of glucagon on mucosal blood flow in the stomach? I am thinking about the difficult problem of gastric erosions, and wondering if glucagon would be helpful in this connection.

Skucas: It is my impression that glucagon decreases mucosal blood flow considerably, while increasing the blood flow to the muscle areas. This is true, is it not?

Jaspan: I cannot answer that from personal experience. I know that it increases portal blood flow at the main vessel level, but I do not know about the mucosal and sub-mucosal levels. I think it is an important question.

Skucas: I believe it does. I mention this partly in reply to Professor Hardcastle's question, and partly because I have heard it suggested that glucagon might be useful in the case of the patient who comes in bleeding from haemorrhagic gastritis; angiography is performed, and there is diffuse oozing throughout. What are you going to do then? The suggestion is that glucagon might be helpful, the idea being to infuse it intra-arterially directly into the vessels feeding the stomach. I have heard this possibility being spoken about, but I do not think I have heard of it actually being tried yet.

Diamant: No, neither have I, but it is an interesting thought.

Hardcastle: Would one need a direct intra-arterial line? Would intravenous therapy not work just as well?

Vilardell: I think it would. I understand that the intra-arterial route has not been found to be particularly advantageous over the intravenous one as far as vasopressin is concerned. I would imagine that the situation is probably about the same in the case of glucagon.

Christiansen: Yes, I agree. I would think that the intravenous route would be quite suitable. Glucagon has the same acid inhibitory effect as intravenous cimetidine, but whereas cimetidine may increase the blood flow, glucagon reduces it. Theoretically, therefore, glucagon could well be effective in this situation.

Vilardell: Would you then go as far as to use glucagon as a prophylactic measure against bleeding in acutely ill patients? I think not, personally, as I would be afraid of the decrease which would occur in the mucosal blood flow. I am thinking of patients in the intensive care unit who in some centres are now routinely given antacids or cimetidine as preventive treatment against erosions and bleeding. Is this perhaps something for which glucagon could be used?

Jaspan: I would worry about this because of the fact that the portal pressure and the portal flow would increase, and I think that one is usually trying to decrease the portal perfusion pressure, irrespective of what is happening at the gastric mucosal level. There are certain patients, however, those with liver disease associated with hypovolaemia, for instance, in whom there are hepatic lobules and areas which are underperfused. If one was to give glucagon to these patients, one could, theoretically, increase perfusion to these areas. I was just reflecting about the patients who are very sick with liver disease; who then get a little better, start to take food orally, and then seem to pick up quite dramatically. Some of the effects seen in these patients may well be due to a meal-stimulated improvement in portal blood flow, in addition, of course, to the nutritional supplementation, which is important. I am not sure of an easy way to distinguish between the blood flow effects and the other effects, but it is a point which should at least be considered.

Bucher: I do not know if one can extrapolate from the rat in this connection, but in the rat blood flow in the regenerating liver does not seem to be all that important. In the eviscerated animals about which I spoke earlier, there is no portal flow at all. There is nothing but the modest flow from the hepatic artery to keep the whole system going, and yet the liver regenerates very well. Blood flow seems not to be a crucial factor in these animals (Bucher, N. L. R., and Swaffield, M. N. (1975) *Proc. Natl. Acad. Sci. USA*, **72**, 1157).

Christiansen: I would not suggest the use of glucagon as prophylaxis in patients in the intensive care unit, but at my hospital we plan to use it routinely in patients with bleeding gastritis, drug-induced gastritis, for instance. Ivey *et al.* have recently shown that glucagon increases the negative potential difference of the gastric mucosa (Ivey, K. J. *et al.* (1980), *Gut*, **21**, 3). What happens in aspirin-induced bleeding gastritis, is that this potential difference is decreased. There were, therefore, good theoretical reasons to presume that glucagon would be effective in this situation.

Vilardell: Let us now discuss the colon. I suppose I am being unrealistic in hoping that glucagon will help in cases of irritable colon.

Hardcastle: In my opinion there are some important questions, particularly with regard to long infusions of glucagon, which have to be answered before we can say how effective this substance is likely to be in the colon. We have to know, for example, for how long its effects can last, how speedily they actually wear off, whether they will come back after a little while, and so on. Only then will one be able to say whether it is likely to be helpful in, for instance, protecting an astomosis by reducing pressure, or in connection with the so-called 'irritable bowel syndrome'. This. incidentally, is a term which I dislike very much. This and 'colon disease' are such mixed bags of problems. It seems very important to me that the patients' problems should be defined more carefully, and that one should know exactly what one is trying to treat.

Vilardell: I agree with you entirely. One sometimes finds even within one hospital department that 'irritable colon' means different things to different physicians. Is there anything more to be said in connection with the colon at the moment?

Miller: I should like to mention just one thing. There is a procedure sometimes used for extracting foreign bodies from the esophagus, also from the rectum of children, and from the biliary tree, whereby one passes a Fogarty balloon up beyond the foreign body, inflates the balloon, and extracts the object in that way. The use of glucagon could well simplify this procedure.

Daniel: Mechanical obstruction is occasionally due to the impaction of a sizeable gallstone just above the ileo-caecal valve. Is it possible that a little glucagon could be of help here by relaxing the spasm of the ileo-caecal valve sufficiently to allow the stone to pass in a natural way?

Miller: Frankly I doubt it. It can, however, be of great help in locating gallstones for the surgeon during the radiology examination. According to the surgical literature, gallstones are supposed to impact in or near the ileo-caecal valve, but I have found them in the right upper quadrant, the left upper quadrant, the left lower quadrant, in fact, more often away from the ileo-caecal valve than near it.

Vilardell: Maybe we should now move on, and discuss the biliary tract. Professor Hardcastle, do you wish to say anything about this?

Hardcastle: Not for the moment, I think. I would rather wait for the results of the double-blind trial we are doing at present on biliary colic before drawing any final conclusions.

Okuda: We know that in animals bile flow increases when there is an increase in portal blood flow. The same thing is probably true for man, but has anyone actually measured portal blood flow in man and recorded the changes which occur after the administration of glucagon?

Jaspan: It is a very difficult thing to measure. At the present time the portal blood flow can, in fact, generally only be measured indirectly. The technique used involves the use of a dye, indocyanin green. One in fact measures hepatic blood flow and then attributes a fixed proportion of 71 % to the portal vein and 29 % to the hepatic artery. This is fine in the basal state, the post-absorptive state, and so on. The problem arises – and now I am speaking about the dog, and I must say that one does not know if this is a good model or not – when one wants to measure the effect of things which change the blood flow: the effect of, for instance, glucagon or somatostatin, or of a meal. This is because the blood flow of the portal vein and that of the hepatic artery do not change in the same way. The portal flow is very responsive and changes quickly and dramatically, whereas the hepatic artery flow hardly changes at all. This is a point which I am afraid is not always taken into account. Several studies have in fact been conducted without attention being paid to this point, and the result, I am afraid, is that the data are completely invalid. The answer to your question, therefore, is no – as far as I know the actual effect of glucagon on portal blood flow in man has not yet been measured.

Rey: I understand that a technique does in fact exist by which this can be done. There are two reports, one from Sweden and one from the UK, in which radiologists have reported doing it during transhepatic cannulations for bleeding varices (Lunderquist, A. and Vang, J. (1974). *N. Engl. J. Med.*, **291**, 646; Scott, J. *et al.* (1976). *Lancet*, **2**, 53). This is a difficult procedure, I agree, and not something to be undertaken lightly, but it can be done.

Baker: In my opinion studies where you cannulate both the portal vein and the hepatic vein and measure the extraction across the liver are more likely to provide the information you are seeking. One must, incidentally, take care with data obtained intra-operatively, as the system is markedly perturbed when one tries to put a flow probe on during an operation, even the basal state in a healthy person.

Vilardell: Let us now discuss the liver. I must say that, as something of an outsider, I was a little surprised to learn that there is so much to be said about liver regeneration. Would anyone like to make further comments about this, or perhaps about conditions other than acute hepatic failure and alcoholic liver disease in which glucagon could possibly be of value? Are there any other fields which should be explored?

Bucher: What about acute toxic injuries of the liver?

Okuda: They would really be regarded as acute hepatic necrosis, or in some instances as fulminant hepatic failure.

Vilardell: But could one not stratify acute liver injuries in some way, and maybe say that glucagon therapy would be more useful in one sort of condition than in another? I am thinking of halothane hepatitis, for example. Would you think that it would be wise to use a glucagon and insulin infusion prophylactically in someone who has had several anaesthesias with halothane and in whom one was afraid of something going wrong?

Okuda: I must say that, at the present time, I see little use for glucagon as a prophylactic. As far as halothane hepatitis is concerned, the patient usually runs a fever before developing liver failure, and this could be regarded as an indication for treatment with glucagon, but I would not use it prophylactically. Dr Oka has presented data relating to the treatment of patients with acute hepatic failure due to viral hepatitis, drug-induced hepatitis, and so on, but in my opinion even in these cases the main value of this therapy lies in its effect to help the liver cells to regenerate. This is so irrespective of the time at which the therapy is begun. In my opinion this explains why the therapy appears to work better in cases of severe acute liver hepatitis than it does in really severe cases of fulminant hepatitis. Personally I recommend it more for patients who have sustained the initial attack. I use it particularly in the sub-acute type of fulminant hepatitis and hepatic failure. Perhaps controlled trials in these conditions would provide us with some useful information in the future.

Diamant: What about after hepatectomy? Do you think that glucagon would be helpful then, by aiding cell regeneration?

Bucher: I can only tell you that in hepatectomized rats endogenous glucagon production suffices.

Okuda: In Japan we often perform extended hepatectomies in patients with hepatocellular carcinoma, sometimes removing as much as three-quarters of the liver. It could well be that in cases such as these insulin and glucagon would be of benefit.

Bucher: It may, but we could not demonstrate any need for it in rats.

Vilardell: Professor Okuda, are these hepatectomies that you are talking about being performed in livers which are otherwise normal, cases of hepatoma on a normal looking liver, for instance, or are you talking about cirrhotic livers also?

Okuda: I was actually talking of otherwise normal livers, not of cirrhotic ones.

Bucher: I would think that as long as the pancreas is normal one probably does not need to give additional hormones.

Hardcastle: I think that in hepatectomy you probably do not need to do so as long as the rest of the liver is absolutely normal. I was just wondering about cases in which embolization of the hepatic artery is used for extensive secondary tumour of the liver, or, particularly, cases of carcinoid syndrome, where one ligates the hepatic artery. Would some sort of supportive therapy be helpful here, do you think?

Jaspan: I am not sure that the bowel is a good model for hepatic regeneration, but, for what it is worth, I would just mention some work which I did in collaboration with Dr. Holmes, who is now working in Edinburgh. We did some work on the bowel very similar to that done by Dr. Bucher, and we too found that no extra stimulus was needed. We resected small intestine in rats and looked at regeneration. We found that this was maximal, but that it could be inhibited with somatostatin. This, I think, suggests that peptides, possibly a whole host of them, which are inhibited by somatostatin, are operative in the regeneration process, and that as long as one does not interfere with the situation, regeneration occurs pretty well. I do not know, but I imagine that the situation might be the same in the liver.

Baker: This is, of course, a very important point. It might in some patients make the difference between survival and death. We have not had nearly the experience with hepatic carcinoma that the Japanese have had, but we have had an opportunity to observe several patients who have undergone extended hepatic resection and these patients have indeed shown a remarkable ability to regenerate. There are two problems. The first is to know in advance which patients are likely to do well without therapy and which are not. The second problem is to know how to measure and to document any effect which insulin and glucagon therapy might have. It is very difficult at the present time to do this. One cannot, for instance, accurately measure the degree of liver regeneration on a liver scan; one can quantitate it roughly, but not at all precisely. Insulin and glucagon therapy may indeed be helpful in some cases, but it will be hard to prove that fact.

Bucher: A cautionary note should be introduced in the light of our recent findings, which are that when the hepatocytes are in a certain metabolic state brought about by prior nutritional conditioning of the animal, addition of particular substrates to the culture causes glucagon to inhibit rather than enhance DNA synthesis. In view of this reversal of glucagon action, it seems wise to proceed with circumspection until the actions of glucagon are better understood.

Jaspan: Dr. Christiansen, I am very interested in your comments about gastric secretion. The effects which you have reported, which are, you point out, physiologic ones, are a bit different to many of the other things we have heard about today. Do you think that these effects might, in fact, be due to the release of vasoactive intestinal polypeptide, or GIP, or other peptides which themselves inhibit gastric secretion. Do you not think that you may, in fact, be looking at a 'second order' phenomenon, rather than at a direct effect of glucagon?

Christiansen: We know from studies that we have performed in man that VIP and GIP are virtually without effect in gastric secretion in man. We have also studied somatostatin, and found that there is no release of somatostatin by glucagon. At this moment we must still conclude that it is glucagon *per se* which has this anti-secretory effect.

Vilardell: Perhaps at this stage I myself might be allowed to mention a possible use for glucagon. There is a fair amount of evidence pointing to the fact that it does not seem to be of much help in acute pancreatitis. I wonder, however, in view of its effect on the sphincter of Oddi, if it is not possible that it could be of some use in biliary pancreatitis. This is something that I would like to see investigated.

I wonder if we might now speak about the side effects of glucagon, and about contraindications to its use.

Jaspan: In my experience there are very few side effects. Occasionally one sees nausea and vomiting, it is true, but this is invariably due to too high a dose being used. As far as contraindications are concerned, I think the only group to whom it might not be wise to give glucagon are diabetics who are not on insulin, because in these patients it is unlikely that extra insulin will be released when the glucagon is given, and this could result in a compromise of glucose tolerance. There is no problem with diabetics who are taking insulin, because in these patients one can always increase the insulin dose to take care of hyperglycaemia. One would possibly not give glucagon to patients with renal failure; I say 'possibly', because I do not really think that high glucagon levels do very much to the metabolic disturbance. In brief then, in my opinion, in the parameters and areas we have discussed today, glucagon has very few side effects and few contraindications.

Miller: I agree with you. However, I would not regard diabetes as a contraindication; certainly not for an ordinary dose, a 'diagnostic' one. There are however two conditions which I should like to mention in this connection. The first is phaeochromocytoma. In these patients glucagon can quite speedily bring on an hypertensive episode. Perhaps this is not an absolute contraindication, because one can take care of the hypertension; nevertheless, glucagon should be used with great caution in such patients. The other contraindication is islet cell tumour, because here instead of bringing about a rise in blood sugar the glucagon will cause the release of a considerable amount of insulin which will have the opposite effect, a fall in blood sugar. These, in my opinion, are the only contraindications.

From the Chairmen: On this note the discussions came to an end. It had been a long day, and we had been hard-pressed to fit so much in. Speaking for ourselves, we were tired, but refreshed too.

There is much to be said for workshops such as this, for days when one is taken away from the concerns of everyday life and closeted together with a group of strangers, specialists from different disciplines, to discuss one specific topic, and to discuss it in depth. It is a time to consider what is known and, perhaps more importantly, what is not known. It is a time to talk, to listen, and to think; a time to speculate, to muse a little, and to wonder ... and not just in one's own field, but in other people's too, and to have them rummage around in yours. This was the second such meeting to be held to discuss glucagon, and already we are hoping that there will be a third.

195

We very much hope that with the publication of the proceedings of this workshop we can pass on some of the knowledge which we acquired. It is sincerely hoped, moreover, that this will become a two-way exchange of information and opinion, one in which you the reader will wish to join. We would indeed be pleased to hear from you (the addresses of all participants are given at the front of this book) should you have data to report, questions to ask, or opinions to give, for it is in this way that the knowledge of all of us will be enhanced.

A. ORIOL BOSCH
F. VILARDELL

Subject index

197